OKANAGAN UNIV/COLLEGE LIBRARY

02498764

**Analysing Health Policy:
Sociological Approaches**

D1026217

RA 418.3 .U6 G74 1998
Green, Judith
Ar-

OKANAGAN UNIVERSITY COLLEGE
LIBRARY
BRITISH COLUMBIA

Analysing Health Policy:
Sociological Approaches

Judith Green & Nicki Thorogood

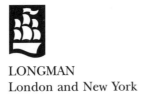

LONGMAN
London and New York

Addison Wesley Longman Limited
Edinburgh Gate
Harlow
Essex CM20 2JE
United Kingdom
and Associated Companies throughout the world

*Published in the United States of America
by Addison Wesley Longman, New York*

© Addison Wesley Longman Limited 1998

The right of Judith Green and Nicki Thorogood
to be identified as authors of this Work has been
asserted by them in accordance with the Copyright,
Designs and Patents Act 1988.

All rights reserved; no part of this publication may be
reproduced, stored in a retrieval system, or transmitted
in any form or by any means, electronic, mechanical,
photocopying, recording, or otherwise without either
the prior written permission of the Publishers or a
licence permitting restricted copying in the United
Kingdom issued by the Copyright Licensing Agency
Ltd., 90 Tottenham Court Road, London W1P 9HE.

First published 1998

ISBN 0 582 29801 6

British Library Cataloguing-in-Publication Data

A catalogue record for this book is available from the British Library

Library of Congress Cataloging-in-Publication Data

Green, Judith, 1961–
    Analysing health policy : sociological approaches / Judith Green,
Nicki Thorogood.
        p.   cm.
    Includes bibliographical references and index.
    ISBN 0–582–29801–6 (paper)
    1. Medical policy—Social aspects—United States.   2. Social
medicine.   I. Thorogood, Nicki, 1964–   . II. Title.
RA418.3.U6G74   1998
362.1—dc21   97–44039
                                                                                    CIP

Set by 35 in 10/12pt New Baskerville
Produced through Longman Malaysia, LSP

Contents

List of boxes

Introduction

Health policy is high on the political agenda in contemporary Britain. It is of concern not only to the policy makers and politicians who decide how the formal health care system is to be financed and delivered, but also to those who work in that health care system, delivering care to the public, and the users and potential users of health care services. 'Health policy' of course also includes a much broader range of issues than those of delivering hospital, community and primary health care services. It is increasingly concerned with the healthy population as well as patients, and with the wider social and physical environments which impact on health. Sociologists have long been interested in health, in its social determinants and health behaviour, and the sociology of health and illness is a thriving subdiscipline. Sociological interest in analysing health policy has perhaps been more recent. Indeed, 'policy-relevant' research has traditionally had a rather ambivalent status compared with more theoretical work within the social sciences. The methods and skills of social scientists have been in much demand to answer questions posed by rapid policy change in the health sector, but applied social research has been seen as low status work, not quite 'proper' sociology. There has been, though, much research in this area which is not only of great potential benefit to policy makers, but which is also theoretically and methodologically interesting for sociologists.

Aim and scope

The aim of this book is to demonstrate the contribution of sociological research to understanding health policy in contemporary

Britain. Throughout, we have made the assumption that 'policy' includes not just the explicit decisions made by government or health authorities, but also the decisions and nondecisions made by all health managers, health professionals and their clients, which constitute policy in its broadest sense.

Using a case study approach, we have taken examples from research done in a range of different settings and for different purposes. The case studies are summaries of published research in the sociology of health and related disciplines, which are used to show how research can illuminate both the policy process itself and its outcomes. We also hope that the material illustrates why sociologists might be interested in health policy as an area of research. Empirical findings related to health policy raise a number of more general issues related to our understanding of social structure and human behaviour, and research in health policy presents methodological challenges for the sociologist.

This is not a comprehensive textbook on health policy, although we have outlined the policy context and debates when relevant and suggested further reading for readers who wish to examine them in more detail. Health policy in Britain is a rapidly changing arena, and many of the contemporary debates described in this book may well be of marginal concern by the time you read it, whereas new ones will have emerged. No textbook on health policy can hope to be up to date by the time it is published, which is why we have focused on approaches to analysing policy, rather than the content of policy itself. The topics selected have arisen from our own experiences of teaching health policy and reflect our own particular areas of interest as well as the analytical approaches we favour. Hopefully, these approaches, and the kinds of empirical work that sociologists engage in, will be of relevance to a range of current health policy problems.

Structure

The material is organised into chapters which introduce four broad areas of health concern: health promotion and public health, primary care, equity in health and health care organisations. Within the chapters, case study examples illustrate various approaches in sociology, and how research contributes to our understanding of the policy process and its outcomes. Inevitably, the divisions between these chapters are rather arbitrary, and there are many cross-references between them.

Chapter 1 introduces health policy analysis, suggests some reasons why health policy has become such a crucial arena for political and social debate since the late 1970s and outlines the potential contributions of sociology to analysing the policy process. Chapter 2 examines the history and growing importance of public health and health promotion in health policy, and links these with theoretical accounts of changing cultural and social formations. Chapter 3 addresses the issue of equity in health as a policy goal, and how sociology has contributed to our understanding of social structural inequalities in access to and outcomes of health care. A consideration of equity in health policy raises contentious issues about rationing and prioritisation. Chapter 4 focuses on research into primary care in the context of calls for a 'primary care-led NHS', where sociologists have been particularly interested in the organisation of general practice, the relationships between professional and patient and, more recently, the question of whether health care is being 'privatised' in Britain. Chapter 5 examines health care organisation, the rise and decline of the hospital and how professionals, managers and patients are affected by organisation. Chapter 6 brings together some of the methodological themes, in exploring some of the practical, political and theoretical issues of concern for sociologists who are doing research into health policy and health services.

Readers unfamiliar with the history and structure of the NHS may want to look at the Appendix first, which provides a brief overview of the history of the NHS and figures showing the main organisations referred to throughout this book.

Acknowledgements

We would like to acknowledge the following people for help, comments and information: Christopher Allen, Naomi Fulop, Charlotte Humphrey, Tim Newton and Pam Smith; and all the students from South Bank University, Guy's Dental School and the intercalated BSc in Sociology as Applied to Medicine who have participated in seminars and discussions over the years.

List of abbreviations

AHA	Area Health Authority
BSA	British Sociological Association
DHA	District Health Authority
DHSS	Department of Health and Social Security
DOH	Department of Health
FHSA	Family Health Services Authority
FPC	Family Practitioner Committee
GMC	General Medical Council
GP	General Practitioner
GDP	General Dental Practitioner
HFA	Health for All
HMO	Health Maintenance Organisation
LA	Local Authority
NHS ME	National Health Service Management Executive
RCT	randomised controlled trial
RHA	Regional Health Authority
STD	sexually transmitted disease
WHO	World Health Organisation

Chapter 1

Health policy and sociology

Summary: Health policy is a key issue of concern to users of health care systems as well as managers, health workers and academics. Economic, ideological and cultural factors contribute to the rising profile of health policy in Britain and internationally. This chapter outlines stages in the policy process, and suggests how sociological research can contribute to an analysis of both the process and its outcomes. Finally it introduces the idea of a sociology of policy, and suggests why sociologists might be interested in an analysis of health policy.

Introduction

It is difficult to avoid debates about health policy in contemporary Britain. As in many other countries, questions about how health care is to be provided, how it is to be paid for and how we can assess its quality, are central to the political agenda. Open any recent newspaper, and the headlines reveal considerable concern with these very questions. Should a girl with leukaemia have her treatment paid for by the health authority, despite low chance of success? Should a popular local hospital close to allow consolidation of services at another site? Is there too much bureaucracy in the National Health Service (NHS)? Should patients be asked to make a payment when they visit their GP?

These issues are no longer of interest just to politicians and the managers of health care services, but also to their users and potential users. They are political questions because they involve value judgements: how do we balance the health needs of individuals against those of the whole population? How far should users' views influence decisions about service provision? To what extent should the NHS be exposed to market forces? The analysis of health policy is, then, a rich field for research. This book aims to outline some of the contributions that sociological research has made to analysing policy in health care. We do not aim to offer a comprehensive description of health policy in modern Britain; there are a number of excellent books available which do this, which you will find listed at the end of this chapter. Neither is this a manual of policy analysis. Again, there are many textbooks which provide thorough accounts of different approaches to policy analysis. Given the rapid changes in policy, we aim instead to describe some tools and approaches which can be used to analyse a number of different issues, and illustrate how they have been used by researchers and policy makers. These tools are, in the main, sociological, although disciplinary boundaries blur when actually doing health care research, and many contributions might owe considerable debts to economic approaches, or social policy ones, for instance. By looking at research on some of the key areas of health care policy in late twentieth century Britain we hope to illustrate how sociological research can help make sense of issues such as why particular developments in policy have happened, what impact they have had on those who use and deliver health care and what an examination of health policy can tell us about wider social change.

The context

A first question might be: why has health policy become such a key political issue in recent years? Policy analysts have offered several answers to this question. Some are economic: they stress the rising costs of the health service, like other parts of the welfare state, and the difficulties that modern governments face in meeting those costs. Other focus more on ideological factors: the changing norms and values in political thought which have altered assumptions about the role of welfare services such as health care in modern society. More recently, sociologists have also been interested in cultural factors to explain the prominence of debates about health. These explanations are clearly interrelated, and a full discussion of the debates about them is outside the scope of this book. However, they form a backdrop to much of the sociological research on health policy, so a brief outline will be worthwhile.

Economic factors

The first set of reasons for the high priority of health policy on political agendas is the rising cost of providing health services for the population. In Britain, spending on health, as well as other welfare services, continued to expand until the late 1970s. Spending on health care did not only grow in absolute terms, but it also grew as a proportion of the nation's income. In 1958 the NHS accounted for about 3.5% of the Gross Domestic Product (GDP), but by 1978 it accounted for about 5.6%. Compared to other health care systems, costs for the NHS are relatively low, but like those in other countries they continue to rise. Table 1.1 shows how health expenditure in Britain compares with other industrialised countries as a proportion of GDP.

Several factors have been suggested to account for these rising health care costs. An initial one is the ageing population profile

Table 1.1 Total health expenditure as percentage of GDP, for selected countries

	1960	1970	1980	1990
Australia	4.9	5.7	7.3	8.2
Denmark	3.6	6.1	6.8	6.3
Germany	4.8	5.9	8.4	8.3
UK	3.9	4.5	5.8	6.1
USA	5.3	7.4	9.2	12.3

Source: OHE 1995

Table 1.2 Population aged 60 and over as a percentage of total UK population

	1971	1981	1991
60+	19.0	20.2	20.7
65+	13.3	15.0	15.7
75+	4.7	5.8	7.8
85+	0.9	1.1	1.6

Source: Grundy 1996

of Britain (see Table 1.2). Rising life expectancy and a falling birth rate mean that a growing proportion of the population is over 60, and a growing proportion of those over 70. Levels of morbidity rise with age, and the health care system has to deal with more chronic disease and long-term care as the population profile ages.

A second factor often cited is increasing demands by users of the health service. After 50 years of the NHS, which provides health care free at point of delivery, it has been argued that generations of patients have grown up with the idea that universal and comprehensive health care provision is a right. The planners of the NHS originally assumed that once urgent health care needs had been met by the new system, demand would start to diminish, as the population became healthier. As Aneurin Bevan suggested:

> the rush for spectacles, as for dental treatment, has exceeded all expectations . . . Part of what has happened has been a natural first flush of a new scheme, with the feeling that everything is free now.
> (A. Bevan 1958; quoted by Klein 1995: 30)

The prediction that costs would decrease as people got healthier proved ill founded, and indeed Bevan's expectation that these high costs were just the initial surge of people getting treatment for eyesight and dental problems for the first time was short-lived. Costs for the NHS continued to rise, and demand for services continued to outstrip supply. Some economists now argue that demand for health care is potentially limitless if there are no reasons to ration that demand. In addition, it has also been suggested that patients are becoming more demanding because of greater knowledge about medicine and health. As people become more informed about health care, and the range of possible interventions, their expectations of what the health care system can offer them rise.

A third reason for expanding health care costs is the constant development of medical technology, such as new equipment and more sophisticated drug treatments. Such developments have increased the number of patients who can potentially benefit from expensive medical intervention. One example is the increasing success of organ transplant operations: between 1979 and 1988, the number of heart transplants in Britain had gone up from three per year to 274 and the number of kidney transplants from 842 to 1,575 (Stocking 1992). Others include the development of intensive care for premature babies and drugs to delay the onset of AIDS in people who are HIV positive.

Given that ability to finance the health care system is not infinite (there is some limit to the amount of taxation that can be levied, although much debate about the level of taxation acceptable), these economic factors raise crucial political questions about health policy. Does the NHS provide 'value for money' compared with other systems? Can some hospital services be provided more efficiently in the community? Should most services remain free at the point of delivery, or should charges be introduced? One contentious issue raised by these considerations of rising costs is the question of rationing. Some 'rationing' inevitably goes on within the NHS: long waiting lists for some operations are, for instance, one way in which health care is rationed. However, this kind of rationing is implicit, and there has been much debate about whether the NHS should explicitly limit either the interventions provided or the groups in the population to whom they are offered. This debate is explored in Chapter 3, in the context of policy which addresses equity in health care.

Although some commentators see these as economic questions which face policy makers in a whole range of health systems, others have focused more on the responses to rising costs, and argued that there are ideological factors which have contributed to the high position of health on political agendas.

Ideological factors

During the 1970s, Britain entered a recession and the conflict between rising demands on the one hand and perceived underfunding of the NHS on the other became critical. Both the professional and public media claimed that the NHS was 'in crisis', indicated by closed wards, health authorities unable to pay bills and problems in nurse recruitment. By the end of the 1970s, the Conservative Party had been elected into office on an explicit platform of encouraging the private market, and bringing in competition to drive down costs in the public sector. In short the political climate became one in which it was possible to question the continued growth in spending on the NHS in the context of 'rolling back the state'. How and why did this happen?

Clauss Offe (1984) provides one account of the decline in consensus around the welfare state, in his arguments about the role of the state in capitalist democracies since the Second World War (see also Chapter 6 for a discussion of differing theories on the role of the state in 'welfare'). Until the 1970s, Offe argues, the welfare state functioned as what he calls the 'peace formula' of capitalist societies. It provided a safety net of assistance and support for citizens who suffered from the risks of capitalism, such as unemployment or health problems. It also recognised a legitimate role for trade unions. This 'peace formula' limited the possibilities for disruptive class conflict. However, from the 1970s onwards, the consensus around the welfare state disintegrated. From the political Right, some critics focused on how the welfare state, with its needs for regulation and relatively high taxation, formed a disincentive to investment. On an individual level, they claimed, the benefits granted by a welfare state lead to a disincentive to work. From the Left were criticisms about the ideological nature of the welfare state and its inefficiencies.

In Britain, the Conservative Party under Margaret Thatcher was a good example of the resurgence of laissez faire ideological ideas, in which the state's commitment to full provision of welfare was being questioned. In terms of health care, perhaps the most influential person on conservative policy was Alain Enthoven, an American health economist, who noted that there were few incentives for efficiency in the NHS. He suggested that such incentives would be provided if hospitals and other health care providers were allowed to compete in a market to provide services (Enthoven 1985). This ideological commitment to using competition as a route to efficiency in health care was translated into the reforms introduced by the NHS and Community Care Act 1990, which set up an 'internal market' in the NHS. The main aims of these reforms were to split the 'providing' and 'purchasing' (or 'commissioning') functions of the NHS. The Appendix shows, in a summarised form, the structure of the NHS after the 1990 reforms and as of April 1996. Health authorities became purchasers of health care for their populations, responsible for assessing the needs of the population and commissioning health services to meet those needs. They could place contracts for these services with private, public or voluntary sector providers. NHS hospitals and providers of community services could become (and the majority did) self-governing trusts, which could raise their own income and capital. Managers of these trusts, who now had to compete for contracts, had an incentive to provide efficient and effective services, and commissioners had an incentive to make the most effective and efficient contracts for their populations. The introduction of fundholding for the larger general practices, which allowed them to place contracts for certain services with hospitals, had a similar aim. The changes to general practice are described in Chapter 4. Overall, the intention was that a 'managed market', or what is sometimes called a 'quasi market' (Le Grand and Bartlett 1993), would replace central planning as the mechanism to control costs.

To what extent was this response to rising costs an inevitable one, and to what extent was it shaped by national politics? As the policy analyst Rudolf Klein notes, 'health care reform was one of the international epidemics of the 1990s' (Klein 1995: 223), and Britain was not alone in attempting radical reforms of its health care system. Most industrialised countries looked at the problem of cost containment, although obviously the solutions they came up with were shaped by national concerns and 'styles' of welfare in their respective countries. What was different about Britain, suggests Klein, was that the British government was rather more successful than others at introducing market-type mechanisms into a public system.

The Conservative administration which introduced market principles into health care had the advantage of a large majority in government, which could legislate radical change without having to make compromises with political opponents. It appears likely that the Labour administration which replaced them in 1997 (with an even larger majority) will maintain the split between the commissioning and provision functions of the NHS. However, there has been considerable debate about the limitations of markets in health care, with commentators pointing to the fragmentation of the NHS (Harrison 1995) and the high costs associated with managing a market (Le Grand and Bartlett 1993). With the return of a government less committed to market principles, the emphasis may change to a more collaborative rather than competitive approach. In addition, political change may change the emphasis of health policy with, for instance, a greater attention to inequalities in health outcomes.

Ideological change, such as that from a postwar consensus about commitment to the Welfare State to a widespread debate on the role of the state, is to some extent the result of this kind of political change at the level of central government, and is perhaps constrained by macro-economic factors such as rising costs. But there are also more diffuse cultural changes in the ways in which 'health' enters the political discourse. These influence the possible solutions that are considered to policy problems (such as the relative emphasis on markets), but they also help shape the very domain of health policy itself.

Cultural factors

Sociologists, in addition to studying the ideological and economic factors, have also considered how these wider cultural shifts that have happened in the late twentieth century have contributed to the focus on health policy. There has been a significant growth in the aspects of our lives that are seen to be related to health. It has been argued that the very domain of health has changed radically over the last two decades:

> Twenty years ago, the mention of health and illness would probably have invoked thoughts of hospitals, doctors, nurses, drugs and a first aid box. Today, however, it would probably conjure up a much broader range of images which could well include healthy foods, vitamin pills, aromatherapy, alternative medicines, exercise bikes, health clubs, aerobics, walking boots, running shoes, therapy, sensible drinking, health checks and more.
>
> (Nettleton 1995: 1)

Rising levels of chronic illness, which is often multifactorial, resulting from lifestyle and environmental factors, rather than the single micro-organisms which cause infectious disease, have shifted the focus of the health service from 'curing' to 'preventing', 'caring' and 'alleviating'. Increasing tranches of social life thus become the concern of health professionals: the amount we drink or eat, our sexual behaviour, our leisure activities. Some sociologists have seen this as a process of the 'medicalisation' of everyday life (Zola 1978), and a result of colonisation by a medical profession anxious to extend the sphere of its influence. Others have focused more on the ways in which health in the late twentieth century has become the concern not only of the medical profession, but of all of us individually. With a change in emphasis from 'curing disease' to 'maintaining health', the health care system has a wide-ranging role in the lives not just of sick people, but healthy populations as well (Bunton and Burrows 1995; Lupton 1995). We do not come into contact with the health services only when we are ill, but are obliged to monitor and manage our own health status in order to stay healthy, by taking exercise, eating the right diet or changing our sexual behaviour. The focus on prevention and health maintenance has been reflected in policy since the late 1970s, when the White Paper *Prevention and Health: everybody's business* (DHSS 1976), which put individual lifestyles firmly on the policy agenda, was published:

> ... many of the current major problems in prevention are related less to man's outside environment than to his own behaviour; what

might be termed our lifestyle. For example, the determination of many to smoke cigarettes in the face of the evidence that it is harmful to health and may well kill them.

(DHSS 1976: 17)

The rise of health promotion and the implications of the emphasis on the individual lifestyle as the object of policy intervention are discussed in Chapter 2.

Given that the domain of 'health' now covers an increasing range of social behaviours, and is one which includes the whole population within its remit, it is perhaps not surprising that policies which impact on health are of key public concern. They do concern all of us, and impact on our lives, whether we see ourselves as ill or healthy.

There are, then, a number of economic, ideological and cultural reasons which contribute to the growing significance of health policy as a cultural and political concern of not just health care professionals, managers and academics, but also of the wider community. Before looking at how sociological research can help our understanding of these changes, we need to define our object of interest: what do we mean by health policy, and how can we analyse it?

What is health policy analysis?

A minimal definition of health policy analysis might be 'The study of health policy concerns, the origins of that policy, its goals and its outcomes'. However, there are many problems with trying to define the field of which health policy concerns might reasonably consist. One often cited definition of health comes from the World Health Organisation: 'Health is not merely the absence of disease, but a state of complete physical, mental, spiritual and social wellbeing' (WHO 1978). The policies which impact on 'physical, mental, spiritual and social well being' are clearly not just those that concern the organisation of health services, but also policies relating to transport, leisure, employment, the role of organised religion and so on. Even if health is more narrowly defined as the 'absence of disease', it is clear that public policy in many different arenas impacts on health. To take just one example, Sonja Hunt (see Box 1.1) looks at the impact of private car use (which is, she argues, outside the traditional remit of health policy) on 'disease, disability, quality of life [and] the integrity of the environment'.

Box 1.1 What should the arena of health policy cover?

Public health has focused on issues of personal lifestyle as
determinants of health status, but the use of private motor cars,
despite having an enormous impact on health, has come in for
little attention. When cars are seen as a health hazard, it is
irresponsible behaviour, such as drinking and driving or not
fastening a seat belt, which has been identified as the public
health problem rather than car use itself.

Road traffic accidents are the fourth leading cause of death
in Britain: on average, 16 people are killed on British roads each
day. They are also the cause of considerable serious disability and
disfigurement. The burden of accidental injury falls most heavily
on the most deprived sectors of society. Boys in social class 5 are
seven times more likely than boys in social class 1 to be killed in
an accident. They are less likely to live in areas with safe places
to play, and more likely to be at risk from traffic travelling fast
through urban residential streets.

In addition to the burden of road traffic accidents, cars have
a range of other serious effects on health. Exhaust emission
increases the concentration of carbon monoxide in the air,
leading to headaches and other symptoms, and other emissions
contribute to cancer and respiratory disease rates. Levels of lead
in the air have been linked to children's development. Driving
itself is a stressful activity with its own direct health costs, as well
as the indirect health costs of discouraging healthy activity such
as walking or cycling.

Sonja Hunt's account of the health impacts of private
motor cars is an indictment of public health for ignoring such
a major cause of death, disability and morbidity in Britain. It also
demonstrates how wide are the range of policies which might
impact on health. Here they include local authority policies
about traffic calming measures, government policies which
encourage or discourage car use; policies which improve
public transport as an alternative; criminal justice policies
which impact on the costs of driving dangerously (such as
penalties for breaking the speed limit) as well as those
policies which concern the treatment and rehabilitation
of accident victims.

Source: Hunt 1989

The boundaries of health policy are, then, blurred at best. Indeed, many recent strategic policy documents recognise this. *The Health of the Nation*, for instance, the 1992 White Paper which set out the Department of Health's targets for improving health in key areas (DOH 1992), advocated the establishment of 'healthy alliances' to work towards targets in local areas (see Chapter 2). These alliances would include representatives from local authorities, and statutory and voluntary agencies as well as the health authority and providers. One of the key areas was accident prevention, and here alliances could usefully include a range of agencies outside the health service, such as the police and fire services, voluntary sector groups involved with children or the elderly, and local schools.

If the field of health policy is difficult to delineate, there are also problems with defining the proper level of analysis: where does policy happen? In her review of the role of sociology in health policy analysis, Margaret Stacey notes that:

> Health policy . . . includes the care and treatment policies developed by consultant clinicians, nurses, midwives and their teams, firms or divisions. It also includes the policies promulgated by general managers, health authorities, the Department of Health and those in charge of private health care arrangements . . . Sociology can be and is applied to policies at all these levels.
>
> (Stacey 1991)

'Policy' does not just consist of national strategic documents such as *The Health of the Nation*, but also how these get implemented by managers, and finally how they are put into practice on the ground, by the health care professionals, patients and wider community who are the object of policy change. The process, of course, also works in the other direction. The range of grounded practices that arise from day-to-day work in the health care sector constitute policy in themselves: they both contribute to the policy agenda and also mould its operation. Thus, the informal practices of the Admission Office clerks studied by Catherine Pope (See Box 5.3 in Chapter 5) constitute 'policy' about waiting lists for operations, as well as government policies such as the Waiting List Initiative. In this book, 'policy' is used in its widest sense, to include all these different levels. To understand how policy is made, and how it impacts on various groups in the population, it is not enough merely to look at the decisions of government departments. We also need to examine the more local arenas of decision making and action.

What can sociology contribute?

To identify how sociology can contribute to policy analysis, it might be helpful to outline the policy process. Policy analysts have written a considerable amount on how to model the policy process, in an attempt to define some common stages through which policies emerge (see, for instance, Hogwood and Gunn 1984). Most frameworks divide the process into a number of chronological subprocesses, such as:

1 *Setting the agenda*   Of the range of problems which face individuals and societies, which ones become selected as 'social problems' and thus become the objects of policy making? How do some of these become seen as the proper domain of health policy? How do demands for action get translated into policy objectives?

2 *Formulation*   How are possible responses to these problems identified? Which groups in society have a legitimate role in forwarding solutions? Who is invited to contribute to the process?

3 *Implementation*   How are policy initiatives decided upon? How are responses by policy makers put into practice at different levels? What are the barriers to the effective implementation of policy?

4 *Evaluation*   What were the outcomes of the policy? Did it meet its explicit objectives? What unintended impacts has it had, and on whom?

Rational or incremental accounts of the process?

Such models suggest that the process is a logical or rational one, whereas in practice policies are likely to be made rather more 'incrementally', by a series of small changes to existing policies, and be the outcome of compromises between various competing interests (Lindblom 1959). It is unlikely that in the 'real world' policy makers are able to assess different solutions to problems and implement them in such a coherent way. Indeed, typically a range of political and other considerations have to be taken into account by policy makers. Given the constraints under which actors within the process work, Lindblom (1959) suggested that the policy-making process was best described as one of 'muddling through' rather than rational planning. Indeed his account of 'incremental planning' is often taken as a prescriptive as well as a descriptive account of policy making: one that outlines how policy ought to be made, as well as how it is made in practice. This is because serious mistakes can be avoided, and policy change is rooted in real problems and their possible and effective solutions, rather than idealistic attempts at the most rational solution. Others claim that as a prescriptive model, Lindblom's incrementalism has an inherently conservative bias: policy merely changes at the margins, but the fundamental principles on which services are provided can never be questioned. One attempt to find a good prescriptive model was Etzioni's idea of 'mixed scanning' (Etzioni 1967), in which fundamental decisions about policy are taken in a 'rational' way, through an exploration of long-term alternatives, whereas detailed policy is made, on the basis of these fundamental decisions, in an incremental way.

Whether rational, incremental or mixed scanning accounts offer the best description perhaps depends on the particular piece of policy making being analysed. It is certainly very rare that policy decisions can be made in a vacuum, without existing structures and vested interests to work with, and even if it were, it would be impossible to examine all possible solutions to the problem. Political interests, cultural values and historical legacies have to be balanced in deciding what policies to implement, and will also influence who is asked to provide possible solutions. Sociological analysis of policy can help examine how those interests operate and what impact they have on policy decisions and nondecisions.

Even if it is limited in describing the reality of policy making, a division of the process into chronological stages does provide a way of thinking about where and how sociology might contribute. Many of these questions about how health policy agendas are set and how solutions are formulated, implemented and evaluated are about social processes. These processes are often planned and intended, such as the introduction of general management into the NHS (see Chapter 5), or the establishment of an internal market. However, there are often unintended or unpredictable outcomes of policy actions as well. It has been argued, for instance, that the introduction of general management also brought with it the unintended consequences of a centralisation of power within the NHS and a decline in the status of nursing (Dopson and Waddington 1996).

Planned change is also implemented against a backdrop of wider social change, which simultaneously facilitates some, and constrains other, policy innovations. Economic factors such as levels of unemployment or cultural shifts in the ways in which we relate to 'experts' such as doctors will impact on the health policy arena.

Sociologists are interested not only in evaluating the planned and unintended outcomes of policy, but also in understanding all parts of the policy process, from the wider social environment of which it is a part to the consequences it has for different groups in the population.

Throughout this book are examples of research which has focused on different parts of the process. The example here is of a study which examined the initial stages of policy making: how are certain issues (in this example, tranquilliser dependence) selected as social problems, and therefore potentially those which come to the attention of policy makers? Michael Bury and Jonathan Gabe focus specifically on the role of the mass media on this process in the study in Box 1.2.

Box 1.2 Why do issues reach the policy agenda?

Background

The perspective employed by Michael Bury and Jonathan Gabe is a 'social problems' approach, which assumes that there is nothing inevitable about the process by which some issues become recognised as 'social problems' worthy of attention. Rather, there are stages by which various groups make claims for the importance of 'their' problem (such as child abuse, gun use, dangerous dogs) and attempt to legitimise some kind of action about that problem. For these claims to be successful, there are certain objective conditions which are necessary (such as evidence of real harm), but not sufficient. The issue examined here is that of the 'excessive' use of legally prescribed benzodiazepines (such Valium and Mogadon), and the role of the mass media in mediating the claims of professional and other groups for policy action.

Although prescriptions for benzodiazepines in Britain have declined from their peak in the 1970s, it has been estimated that about 3% of the population of Britain have used tranquillisers for over a year. Recent concern has been about the effects on these patients, with claims being made in the scientific literature that a large proportion of patients were suffering from dependence and from withdrawal symptoms if they tried to stop.

The study

Bury and Gabe first examined the claims made by medical experts and various mental health pressure groups that benzodiazepines were abused (i.e. prescribed for symptoms which would not benefit from them) and overused. It was claimed that patients were experiencing real problems in trying to withdraw from using these drugs. Reasons given included criticism of general practitioners (GPs) for using repeat prescriptions rather than taking time to talk to patients, or being too influenced by drug company advertising. Such claims were subject to counter claims from other experts, who argued that accounts of withdrawal problems were exaggerated.

The media have a key role both in bringing these claims to the attention of the public, and in shaping the message. Why, then, did the media take up the claims made by these pressure groups and medical experts from the countless claims made by other pressure groups and experts about a whole range of other issues? Several reasons for the resonance of claims with public sensibilities are suggested. First, any issue concerning health is an important one for the modern media, given the expanding interest in the domain. A second is the increasing role of the law as a method of redress for those who have been harmed by medicine. Tranquilliser use was a good example of this, as individual patients have attempted to sue GPs or drug companies to compensate for the harm caused by tranquillisers.

Next, the authors examine in detail how the media shape the message. They take examples of television programmes of different formats, including the popular magazine programme *That's Life!* and the investigative journalism format of *The Cook Report* as examples of two British programmes which have addressed the issue of dependence. Two particular images dominated television coverage. The first was that of the 'distressed woman' at the centre of the story, who was portrayed as an 'ordinary person' with relatively minor problems who had been 'taken over' by drug use and her dependence. The second was of the drugs themselves, shown as abundant and dangerous. Programmes rely on a narrative to tell a good story, and here there are 'victims' who face the 'villains' of the GP and drug companies. The use of benzodiazepines also reflects ambivalences in society in general, about mental health and drug taking. Thus the media can amplify claims made by various groups, as well as legitimating them.

This 'issue' was, then, one which met not only the necessary conditions for a problem to reach the policy agenda (in that there was evidence of real harm) but also met other conditions: it resonated with contemporary social concerns about health in general, about the role of the law in mediating individual complaints about health services and about drug use in particular.

Source: Bury and Gabe 1990

This kind of research on how certain problems become seen as 'policy issues' demonstrates that there is nothing inevitable about how the policy agenda is set. Various interest groups make claims for action, and whether they are successful or not is the result of a range of social and cultural factors, rather than any objective level of need for action. Similarly, if we look at the second stage, formulation, not all possible solutions to the problems will be considered. Again, some groups in society will have more power to identify possible policy actions than others. Changing governments, for instance, will actively seek policy advice from different agencies. The Adam Smith Institute may have more influence with a conservative administration than the Policy Studies Institute. At a more local level, informal professional and social networks may, for instance, influence whether an effective healthy alliance is established, and the shape it takes. The sociologist Ann Greer examined how new medical technologies (such as CT scanners or laser surgery) were disseminated through professional communities, and noted that whether professionals utilised these technologies had very little to do with their 'objective' worth, as measured by scientific reports (Greer 1988). Instead, local communities developed a consensus around whether a technology would be taken up or not, based on whether it was utilised by local 'opinion leaders' and whether it was the kind of thing that 'fitted' with local norms. A similar point could be made about policy change: most requires an element of voluntary change in the implementation phase, and this is unlikely to happen as an inevitable result of evidence that the policy would be effective.

Sociology provides a wide range of tools which can be used to help us address these issues in the production, implementation and evaluation of health policy. Quantitative studies, such as examination of secondary statistics or ad hoc surveys, can aid in evaluating needs for services or the impact of policy on different groups. Qualitative techniques, such as ethnographic studies or in-depth interviews, can illuminate the processes by which policy gets implemented (or not) or how certain problems get selected as worthy of the attention of policy makers. The methodological questions raised by doing research into health policy are brought together in Chapter 6.

As well as drawing on different methods, these studies also have rather different aims. Some were designed to influence policy makers, others were primarily studies in sociology, which have policy implications as an unexpected outcome. Gordon *et al.* (1977)

suggest a helpful distinction between analysis *for* policy, and analysis *of* policy. The former, they suggest, would include activities such as policy advocacy and the provision of information, such as demographic information, to policy makers. The latter would include analysis of the policy process itself and the analysis of outcomes of policy. Evaluation and policy monitoring could be either, depending on its aim. The crucial distinction is perhaps who the analysis is for: whether the agenda and goals are set by the policy makers, or by the analysts themselves. A similar distinction could be made for the contribution of sociology. The questions addressed by sociological researchers in health policy could be divided into two overlapping sorts: those which contribute to an analysis *for* policy and those which contribute to an analysis *of* policy.

- Sociology for policy aims to provide research findings which improve the policy-making process or its outcomes. It is often 'prescriptive' in that it makes explicit recommendations.
- Sociology of policy is done to understand what health policy is: what its role is, how wider social and cultural forces impact on its form and content and how an examination of health policy can inform us about the society that produced it.

The final sections of this chapter outline examples of these different enterprises.

Sociology for health policy

One motive for sociological research in health policy is to have some impact on the policy process: to provide data or ideas which will influence policy makers, and improve either the process of policy making or its outcomes. The key questions for a sociology for health policy are: what should health policy look like, and how should it be implemented? Research for health policy is done in a number of settings including academic departments, where the results are usually published in refereed journals, and within health agencies, where research is specifically commissioned to inform the policy process. Here, results may be disseminated more locally, in what is known as 'grey literature', the in-house reports which go to managers in a position to implement recommendations, but may not have a wider circulation (see Box 6.1 for an example).

At first sight, it is difficult to find examples of sociological research having any direct and demonstrable impact on policy formation. It is rather easier to cite examples of where research has been ignored. The Report of the Working Group on Inequalities in Health (better known as the Black Report, after its chair, Sir Douglas Black) is one instance (Townsend and Davidson 1982). The committee was charged with the task of collating information about differences in health status between occupational groups in Britain, examining the factors which contribute to these differences and assessing the policy implications. Their findings are now well known: that at all stages in the life cycle, health experiences were poorer for the lower occupational groups, and that factors in the socioeconomic environment were likely to be a major cause of those differences. Their policy suggestions were wide-ranging, including a number of measures to provide children with a better start in life, such as free school meals, day care facilities, increases in child benefit and maternity grants as well as suggestions about direct health care provision. The impact of these conclusions on the policy agenda are also well known: they were rejected wholesale by the then Secretary of State, Sir Patrick Jenkin. He argued that the costs of instituting such a programme were unrealistic, and that the validity of the committee's findings was in doubt. Despite provoking widespread public and academic debate, the report had little immediate impact on policy making.

Even when research has been commissioned by users of services specifically to inform policy, the results can have unexpected impacts. Claudia Martin (1988) describes how a survey of consumer satisfaction with maternity services in the Lothian area of Scotland was commissioned by a pressure group concerned about possible closures of local maternity units. The report was leaked to the press, and various parties made selective use of the results to justify their preferred policy option. For the Health Board, concerned to cut costs and centralise services, the findings that women were equally satisfied in all hospitals was used to justify the planned closure of one unit. For the pressure group, it was used to justify maintaining local choice for women. Despite having had little impact on the decision on hospital closure, Martin argues that this kind of research still has beneficial effects on policy making. In this case, she says that one outcome was that the Health Board had to take public opinion into account in further planning, and did have some data to draw on to inform them of clients' views.

Such examples should not, then, lead to pessimism about the possible influence of sociological research for policy. As Bulmer (1982) points out, looking for evidence of direct influence assumes a rather linear relationship between research and policy, with the researcher conceived of almost like an 'engineer', who provides information that fits neatly into the gaps identified by policy makers. A more realistic model of how research impacts on policy, he suggests, is that of 'enlightenment', in which sociological research contributes to the cultural backdrop against which policy is constructed. So, for instance, work such as that of Erving Goffman (1961) on 'total institutions', although not designed narrowly as 'policy research', had an impact through its contribution to changing social ideas about the role of the hospital in treating mental illness, which formed part of the 'cultural backdrop' to the NHS and Community Care Act (see Chapter 5). In the case of the Black Report, even though the government chose not to implement the recommendations, there were significant gains made in the longer term. Richard Wilkinson, for instance, notes how research like this has gradually shifted public opinion on the importance of economic conditions to health, which will eventually force political change:

> [There has been an] extraordinary increase in public awareness of health inequalities . . . over the last twenty years. Initially, when the subject of social class differences in death rates came up in conversation with doctors and others involved in healthcare, the first question was usually to ask which way round the differences were . . . Since then, the relationship between poverty and poor health has become common knowledge . . . This transformation of public awareness has come about as the result of the repeat coverage by the media of a constant stream of research findings on numerous different aspects of the size and causes of health differences.
>
> (Wilkinson 1996: 231)

Often, it will be impossible to trace the origins of a particular change in the orientations of policy makers. After all, researchers and policy makers do not work in completely autonomous spheres, and they may share overlapping influences. Virginia Berridge and Betsy Thom discuss these 'policy communities' as a way of understanding the relationship between research and policy in the areas of drug use in Box 1.3.

Box 1.3 Policy communities: the relationships between research and drug policy

Virginia Berridge and Betsy Thom outline various models which have been suggested for the relationship between policy and research. One concept they find useful is that of 'policy communities', which are the groups of central policy makers and the agencies with which they have close relationships. Whether research knowledge is utilised at particular times by these communities is the result of various economic, social and political forces. They draw on published research and policy documents as well as interviews with key actors in the process (such as researchers and civil servants) to examine the relationship between research and policy.

From this data they trace the particular constellation of forces which have influenced research and policy in the areas of drug and alcohol use and smoking and lung cancer. The case study of drugs research illustrates how policy communities shape the influence of research. One study which was widely cited as influential in changing drug policy was a trial of heroin and methadone prescribing in the late 1970s. The results of this study suggested that prescribing heroin to drug users increased the tendency for them to carry on using drugs, but decreased the risk of them engaging in criminal activity. Despite this ambivalent conclusion, Berridge and Thom argue that the papers resulting from this study were used as scientific justification for shifting drug policy away from maintenance doses and towards the advocacy of short-term methadone prescribing, with eventual abstinence as its aim. It appears that this research did not inform policy, but acted as a post hoc rationale for it. Some of the reasons contributing to this lie in the position of medical doctors within the newly established drug dependency units. To be merely dispensing maintenance doses clearly had less prestige than managing active treatment, such as methadone as part of a withdrawal programme. The political influence of these doctors meant that a policy of maintenance was less likely to be advocated.

Other changes to drug policy – such as the introduction of needle exchanges in the 1980s – utilised research in a similar way. Here, argue Berridge and Thom, there had been a strong consensus among researchers that 'harm minimisation' (reducing the impact that drug use has on other areas of life, such as health or criminal activity) was a more reasonable policy goal than trying to eliminate illicit drug use completely. The change from an abstinence model was partly a reflection of shift towards a less medical focus within the policy community, which by the 1980s included a broader range of professional views, such as those of voluntary agencies and social scientists. However, schemes such as needle exchanges, which enable injecting drug users to get clean needles and so reduce the risk of infections, remained controversial. Only when the issue of AIDS and HIV infection became a political crisis was it possible for this community to influence policy change, and the Department of Health commissioned research specifically to evaluate needle exchange schemes. Before then the political policy of a 'war on drugs' made any harm minimisation interventions politically unacceptable. The important links in this policy community are those between medical civil servants and the politicians.

That these links were crucial is illustrated by the contrasting example of the fate of needle exchange research in New York City, which did not have a similar policy community with a consensus around goals and how to achieve them. Although researchers in New York did have some success at setting up an evaluation of a needle exchange scheme, this had to be set up as a scientific experiment rather than a policy evaluation, and remained solely in the sphere of research, rather than policy. In New York City, there was opposition from the health community itself, the police and also black and Hispanic politicians, who saw 'harm minimisation' policies as racist, in that they did not address prevention of drug misuse within their communities. Without the establishment of a policy community, with effective links with politicians and a consensus about response, the research failed to impact on policy.

Source: Berridge and Thom 1996

The impact of sociological research on policy may, then, be rather difficult to untangle, as the direction of influence is rarely linear. As Mel Bartley (1994) notes, in her study of the relationship between research and policy on unemployment, to ask 'how does research impact on policy?' is really the wrong question, as the two are intertwined processes. Policy agendas influence the kinds of research which is undertaken, and sociology has diffuse and (sometimes) unpredictable effects on the processes it seeks to describe and analyse.

The sociology of health policy

This section takes a different perspective, and, rather than examining the ways in which a sociological approach can *enhance* the formation and implementation of health policy, it analyses the *concept* of Health Policy from a sociological perspective.

Health policy is a relatively new invention. Prior to the last half of the nineteenth century it would not have been possible to think in terms of developing state policies in relation to many areas which we now completely take for granted: housing, education, poverty, employment, health. Indeed it is these domains, which came into existence a little over a century ago, that now constitute the realm of a broad-based 'social policy'.

It should be noted that the end of the nineteenth century saw the widespread application of 'scientific reasoning', the growing dominance of medical science and the increased dependence on 'statistics' (see also Chapter 6), that is, the notion that abstractions can have rates and trends and properties, such as the birth rate or the death rate of a population. As well as becoming a central tool of government, this was also held to offer great promise to the practice of medicine. Nineteenth century statisticians were optimistic about the role of numbers in improving medicine. William Farr, the first statistician to the Registrar General, wrote:

> Medicine, like other natural sciences, is beginning to abandon vague conjecture where facts can be accurately determined by observation; and to substitute numerical expressions for uncertain assertions . . . the physicians of this century will be saved from the fallacies of partial generalisation.
>
> (Registrar General 1839: 63)

This historical moment also heralded the colonisation and mapping of previously uncharted territories: the great urge towards taxonomy and classifying and the birth of the 'detective' and the detective genre of fiction (for example, Wilkie Collins' book *The Moonstone*, first published in 1868 and widely regarded as the first detective story, and Conan Doyle's 'Sherlock Holmes' stories published between 1887 and 1927). The possibility existed for the revealing of truth by the ordering, observing and analysis of signs or clues as a means of detecting underlying causes. This was a new way of making sense of the world and one strand was the notion of a public health which could not only be uncovered and charted but directed and influenced (see Chapter 2). The existence of a policy for health will therefore tell us something about the priorities and values of the society that produces it. Currently any policy relating to 'health' locates health within a medical discourse. Thus 'health' is constructed through scientifically defined criteria which can be measured and, in theory at least, achieved. Health is part of the new scientific paradigm and health policy part of the social domain.

How we can we account for this positioning? What is it that links the scientific-medical discourse of health with the domain of the social? There are a number of differing theories, both sociological and not (e.g. historical), which can be offered as explanatory frameworks (see Chapter 6), but it is our intention here to take a social constructionist perspective which steps back and asks how a field of health policy could have emerged in the way it did. One writer who has had a significant impact on this kind of approach is the French philosopher Michel Foucault, whose analysis has been a productive starting point for many sociologists of health policy.

From a Foucaultian perspective these two domains are linked by the emergence of the concept of *the population* (with its statistical properties such as birth rates and death rates, for example) and this in turn creates the space for the emergence of public health as a discourse. In other words, shifts during the nineteenth century, such as the growth of statistics, are facets of a changing discourse, which makes it possible to speak about 'public health' as a discrete activity. How 'health' is achieved on a population-wide, rather than individual basis becomes the grounds for the formulation of 'health policy' and creates the domain of the 'social'.

These notions, according to Foucault, indicate a shift away from a prenineteenth century understanding of power which was exercised by the sovereign (king) through the (male) 'head of the family' towards a more subtle form of the play of power. This is exercised through 'the population' and those segments of it – individuals, families and communities – which constitute it but no longer represent it. This knowledge pertaining to the population, its patterns and statistics is central to the project of 'public health' and to the new techniques of power identified by Foucault (1979) as discipline and surveillance. Thus a Foucaultian analysis suggests that a discourse such as 'public health' can only emerge within a disciplinary society. For Foucault, the health of the population as a whole becomes a legitimate object of government, to be achieved:

> Either directly through large scale campaigns or indirectly through techniques that will make possible, without the full awareness of the people, the stimulation of birth-rates, the directing of the flow of population into certain regions or activities etc.
>
> (Foucault, quoted in Burchell *et al.* 1991: 100)

Government, through public health, is therefore interested in describing the lives and health of the population. Health policy constructs that domain.

What then have been the objects of health policy? Historically we have seen the object of 'health' split between the individual (subject to the routines and discipline of hospital or GP and situated in the 'institution') and the population, subject to discourses of hygiene and prevention and situated in the 'community' (Armstrong 1993). Each could be used to chart changes in 'social priority' through time. As Foucault says: '. . . political practice did not transform the meaning or form of medical discourse, but the conditions of its emergence, insertion and functioning; it transformed the mode of existence of medical discourse' (Foucault, quoted in Burchell *et al.* 1991: 67). Thus 'health' is a site of discipline and surveillance, whether that be within a hospital (where the receipt of care is dependent on the patient's obligation to be examined 'right up to death', Foucault, in Burchell *et al.*: 67); at a population level, through epidemiology; a particular way of documenting sickness as disease categories; or through categories of health and disease becoming part of the system of administration and political control of the population.

Health policy has been the site of regulation on the basis of many arenas of contemporary social tension, for example, on the basis of race, often expressed as a fear of 'infection' (both literally and metaphorically) by the foreigner whether it is centred on monitoring TB at the point of immigration or the taking over of 'our' corner shops. Health policy also operates on the basis of gender: the medicalising of child birth, the regulation of 'families' through welfare interventions (Donzelot 1980, Bloor and McIntosh 1990); and perhaps more obviously, on age: the reissue of driving licences depend on the physical capacity of older people, the prescription of contraceptives for girls and women, which are strictly regulated on the grounds of age (Hawkes 1995). The sites in which health policy operates can give us insight into the values and preoccupations of the contemporary 'social arena', and 'health' can often be the justification offered for what Stan Cohen (1973) called 'moral panics' (for example, issues as diverse as AIDS/HIV, 'raves' and the ownership of pit bull terriers).

The arena of public health and health promotion is a good example of a domain of health policy which has been addressed by sociologists interested in accounting for its emergence and what its form and content reveal about wider social and cultural change. The following chapter will consider how public health and health promotion construct aspects of social life.

Exercises

Exercise 1

Clip out all the reports which deal with health care or health policy from a national or local daily paper for one week. As well as in the current affairs pages and specialist health sections carried by some national newspapers, you may find health covered in 'lifestyle', problem pages or other sections.

To what extent do they deal with:

• advice on personal health care?
• reports on strategic health policy (such as government white papers, health care reforms nationally and internationally)?
• reports on the implementation of health policy (such as decisions by local health authorities)?
• advances in medical knowledge?

As a seminar exercise, compare the coverage of the newspaper you looked at with coverage in other newspapers looked at by the group.

Exercise 2

A recent judicial challenge may mean that (expensive) drugs therapy for HIV/AIDS must be made available in all health authorities where it is required, regardless of cost.

Try to identify the economic, political and cultural debates for and against this policy change.

Exercise 3

Using a current newspaper or news broadcast identify how many 'stories' have recourse to using 'health' as a justification for whatever action is being proposed. Can you find any issues in which competing claims both use 'health' as a basis for their argument (e.g. the issue of condoms to prisoners)?

Further reading

Introductions to policy analysis
Ham, C. and Hill, M. (1993) *The Policy Process in the Modern Capitalist State,* Hemel Hempstead: Harvester Wheatsheaf.

A good introduction to theoretical accounts of the policy process, which examines theories of the state, the role of bureaucracy, power and the study of organisations.

General accounts of health policy
Walt, G. (1994) *Health Policy: An Introduction to Process and Power,* London: Zed Books.

A comprehensive and readable overview of health policy analysis, outlining the main debates and drawing examples from an international perspective.

On modern British health policy
Allsop, J. (1995) *Health Policy and the NHS: Towards 2000* (2nd edn), Harlow: Longman.
Ham, C. (1992) *Health Policy in Britain* (3rd edn), London: Macmillan.
Ranade, W. (1994) *A Future for the NHS? Health Care in the 1990s,* Harlow: Longman.

These three texts provide a thorough account of the development of health policy in Britain in the second half of the twentieth century, and of the major issues of concern to contemporary policy makers.

On the sociology of health policy
Gabe, J, Calnan, M. and Bury, M. (1991) *The Sociology of the Health Service,* London: Routledge.

This is one of the few collections which analyses issues in health policy from sociological perspectives. Chapters on privatisation, professional power, management, evaluation, general practice, health promotion and community care demonstrate sociological and multidisciplinary perspectives within the health services.

Chapter 2

Public health and health promotion

Summary: The predominant themes of public health during the nineteenth century may be broadly summarised into three main periods: sanitation, with a focus on drains and dustbins; contagious diseases, as part of a discourse of moral regulation; and 'lifestyle and behaviour', with the emphasis on individuals and their culture.

This chapter examines the emergence of public health during the latter part of the nineteenth century and its consequent development into the current discourse of the 'New Public Health'. There is a summary of what kinds of policy are produced by these practices and a discussion of them as examples of disciplinary power. This debate is extended with a consideration of the theory and practice of health promotion and the related issue of 'risk' and 'risk assessment'. The chapter ends with a discussion of the most recent function of public health, that is, community needs assessment.

Introduction

Initially, the newly fledged 'public health' of the late nineteenth century was concerned with 'drains, dustbins and diseases' (*Critical Public Health* 1992) and was known as the Sanitary Reform movement. This early public health movement emphasised what are now known as environmental issues, such as clean water, sewers and housing conditions. An example of these early (public) health policy concerns were the activities of the General Board of Health during 1848–75 when Ernest Chadwick, as head, campaigned for sanitary reform emanating from the achievement of the first National Public Health Act in 1848.

Alongside this 'environmental' approach to the monitoring and regulation of health was another developing perspective, that of the medical (see Chapter 1). In 1854 a new post, that of Medical Officer of Health, was created. Chadwick was deposed and replaced by John Simon, who was the first 'medical man' to hold government office. Considerable conflict took place between the two perspectives, but by 1870 sanitary engineering was superseded by 'sanitary science' which was premised on a more individualistic perspective derived from the new 'germ theory' of disease. This emphasised immunisation, vaccination and other personal preventive services.

In public health's own story, its birth is generally regarded as the moment when John Snow halted the Soho cholera epidemic in 1854 by removing the handle of the Broad Street water pump. A shortened version of the story is as follows. There was an outbreak of cholera in a particular area of London; many died within this fairly small contained area but no one knew why. It transpired, however, that two cases, and only two, had been identified in the far-removed district of Hampstead. At this time dominant theoretical paradigms looked to bad air, miasma, produced from the piles of putrefying rubbish which accumulated in the heavily populated central areas. John Snow, however, made the revolutionary move of plotting these cases on a map, and followed it up by seeking out information on the preceding activities of the two affected women in Hampstead. What he was to discover was that they had recently left the Soho district and, having particularly enjoyed the water from this area, were having it bottled and brought to Hampstead. Thus, Snow deduced, the water was to blame although no one knew quite why. However removing the pump handle, that is, stopping the source of the disease, had the desired effect of stopping the outbreak of any more cases.

This account has a number of significant elements. First, John Snow was a physician, marking the moment at which it became legitimate for a medical doctor to take interest in affairs of public life. Secondly it was possible to conceive of such an entity as public life. These two conditions produced the third significant element: the adoption of an *epidemiological* approach, that is the plotting of the incidence and the prevalence of disease in a social space. Finally, the stop-it-at-source approach of public health was born.

The shift from the sanitary reform to the sanitary science perspective demonstrates a shift from a lay/structural to a medical/individual perspective. The prevention of ill health became a professional activity, requiring the skills of doctors, and one which focused on the behaviours of individuals rather than the conditions in which they lived. However, what both perspectives have in common is that they imply a reservoir of disease constantly present in the community. The new thinking, however, believed the presence of disease to be a normal part of the social world (rather than the wrath of God, for instance) which must, nevertheless, be monitored in order to be able to control and prevent it.

As mentioned in the Introduction, the latter half of the nineteenth century saw the emergence of new forms of power; those of routine monitoring and surveillance. Policy formation produced by the new political practices took place in a number of arenas we now know as 'social', for example, public education, housing, standing armies, large institutional hospitals and prisons (this is discussed further in Chapters 5 and 6). Public health fits right into this model of discipline, monitoring and surveillance: it constantly surveys a healthy population with the aim of preventing disease. These are not necessarily conscious or explicit techniques imposed 'from above' with the aim of maintaining social order. They are, however, practices which become part and parcel of our daily lives, rules which we choose to obey. These kinds of practices are often 'for our own good' and involve self-monitoring and self-discipline (e.g. Foucault's (1979a) description of Bentham's model of the Panoptican, again see discussion in Chapter 5).

Social regulation has often been achieved through the use of routine practices and hygiene rules, for example those of monastic orders. But with the increase in population during the last half of the nineteenth century these techniques formed the new political practices. As Nettleton (1992) has pointed out, the discursive practices of dentistry are a good example of this model. In 1870 the Compulsory Education Act made it possible to carry out the 'toothbrush drill' in schools; this involved rows and rows of children in a daily demonstration of tooth brushing technique, monitored and surveyed by the 'expert', by which actions they hoped to instil a lifetime of 'good practice'. Indeed, schools remain the site of statutory medical and dental surveillance, although the content of these activities may have changed.

'Public health' has a number of distinct discursive practices. It has become the epidemiological branch of medicine, concerned with classifying disease, establishing aetiology and recommending medical intervention to prevent the occurrence of disease. Public health has also incorporated notions of the ecological and social context of health. The object of these new technologies is the spatial relationships, both social and geographical, between institutional bodies (Armstrong 1993) and individual bodies, which can be schooled, shaped, manipulated by the practices of current health policy.

Clearly health policy, which has created as its object the subjective human body, will be centrally involved in producing this. 'Hospital medicine' is employed in the repair and correction of such things that escape the public health net and it is not therefore surprising that public health should be concerned with the routine surveillance of bodies and the promotion of 'healthy behaviours'.

The practices of public health medicine and dentistry over the last 100 years have been well documented (Nettleton 1992, Armstrong 1983, Mort 1987). These can be broadly described in terms of three shifts in focus: having begun with a solely environmental focus (sewers, drains and housing) there came the first shift, to the epidemiological phase, with child health surveillance, contact tracing and the 'dispensary' (Armstrong 1983). This phase focuses on the interaction of the body, or the mouth, and the environment. Subsequently came the addition of the psychological phase. This concerned itself with the relationship between the body or mouth and the mind. It was no longer enough simply to document the existence of disease, it became important to understand why people persist in what are deemed unhealthy behaviours. Thus the psychological concepts of pain, stress and anxiety are employed to help understand and explain these human phenomena. These techniques also inform health promotion and education strategies: advising how best to reach the people deemed in most need of education, or determining the most effective techniques for changing people's behaviour. This approach tries to answer why it is that, despite everything they know about the health hazards, some people still eat sugar (for example).

The third shift is to the 'social'. It becomes apparent that these individual psychological traits do not occur at random, that there are underlying unifying factors leading to, for example, high sugar consumption or failure to attend for smear testing. Instead it is the values and attitudes of the people concerned which serve to produce the framework for their behaviour. Public health now seeks the origin of medical and dental problems in the social domain: in the population characteristics of socioeconomic class, culture, gender, race, disability and sexuality:

> the very essence of the patient's individuality, however, is influenced by his environment and therefore it is important not only to think of a patient as a person, but also in the context of the community. The appalling record of dental health in this country is in part due to the result of treating patients without reference to the influences of the environment in which they live and work. An essential part of sociology teaching is that some of an individual's attitudes and behaviour cannot be understood without reference to his collective existence. *We cannot treat individuals as isolated units. A person visiting his dentist takes with him a set of learned beliefs, values, symbols from his own social world.*
>
> (Blinkhorn 1979: 118, emphasis added)

In the second half of the twentieth century we have witnessed a return to the more traditional nineteenth century public health approaches, with concerns about structure, environment and ecology. A broader approach has become apparent in physical medicine where the focus has been on the individual within his or her own psychosocial context. Lifestyles and behaviour have become concerns of public health and clinical medicine. Dentists and doctors are no longer dealing with a set of parts but with a whole person. Suddenly under scrutiny is exactly what we do in the bedroom, bathroom, kitchen and supermarket as well as in school.

Before exploring further the rise of health promotion and education as the dominant arm of contemporary public health, we first turn to the development of what has become known as 'the New Public Health'.

The 'New' Public Health and health education

During the 1980s a new model gained currency, now known as 'the New Public Health' (Ashton and Seymour 1988). Leading proponents of this approach were John Ashton and Howard Seymour, who as Senior Lecturer in Community Health at Liverpool University and Regional Health Promotion Officer for the Mersey Regional Health Authority respectively, were the architects of the 'New Public Health' strategies developed in Liverpool during the 1980s.

This model attempts to integrate the dual medical/social aspects and to pick up on the 'progressive' critique of traditional health education methods coming from within the discipline and from community development. The New Public Health rhetoric draws on the World Health Organisation's broad definition of health and the 'Health For All' (HFA) programme of intersectoral responsibility and public participation.

This New Public Health sees as its legitimate object areas of public life previously marginalised or excluded. It should now be addressing, amongst others, economic, political and environmental targets, not limiting itself to the social/medical. Thus public health could be regarded as having returned to its roots in the Sanitary Reform movement. This is not without irony for the present day (local authority) environmental health officers who feel that this is what they have been saying and doing all along, but without the benefit of either a medical degree's status or indeed its salary! (Acton and Chambers 1990).

The history of public health is also a history of local government, as responsibility for public health has been bounced back and forth between health service and local authority control. It has been noted earlier that 'health' has been produced by the creation of the 'social domain' and that the presence or absence of health is more likely related to the activities in these other, social, spheres, for example, education, law, housing, than to the existence or implementation of a 'health' policy. Indeed until recently (1974) these areas were the remit of local government, at least as far as local policy formation and implementation were concerned (see Table 2.1).

One consequence of this close rivalry or alliance (depending upon your viewpoint) has been a number of joint working practices. A chronology of the changing policy-making bodies would soon date; thus this chapter is more concerned with analysing the changing *processes* which constitute health policy and which illuminate the key issues.

A central theme has been the commitment by health authorities and local authorities to the WHO 'Health For All (HFA) by the year 2000' targets (WHO 1985). This will be discussed in more depth in Chapter 4, but the study in Box 2.1 illustrates some of the issues raised by a more collaborative approach to public health.

Table 2.1 A summary of key dates in the history of 'Public Health'

1832	Reform Act (Poor Law Commission with Chadwick as Secretary).
1836	Registrar General established (thus the first recording of 'population statistics').
1842	Report on the Sanitary Condition of the Labouring Population of Great Britain: Chadwick's report which led to the rise of the sanitary movement.
1848	1st Public Health Act.
1848	Appointment of John Simon as Medical Officer of Health.
1866	Sanitary Act: placed local authorities under obligation to inspect their district.
1868	Housing Act: local authorities could ensure owners kept properties in good repair.
1871	Local Government Board Act, became Ministry of Health in 1919.
1872	Public Health Act: made Medical Officer of Health compulsory.
1875	Public Health Act: increased powers of local authorities and brought together all aspects of public health law. Local Authorities to establish their own sanatoria.
1902	Midwives Act: licensed midwives now employed by local authorities under the Medical Officer of Health.
1906	Education (provision of meals) Act: school dinners.
1907	Education (administration) Act: began the School Medical Service.
1907	Notification of Births Act: provided the space for the creation of health visitors.
1913 & 21	Local Authorities responsible for providing treatment for VD and TB.
1918	Maternity and Child Welfare Act: local authorities responsible for routine check-ups and surveillance.
1929	Local Government Act: transferred some hospitals into direct local authority control.
1936	Public Health Act: consolidated the public health functions and the personal and clinical services provided by the local authorities.
1942	Beveridge Report: identified the five giant evils: want, disease, ignorance, squalor and idleness.
1946	NHS Act: removed all clinics and dispensaries from local authorities and established separation of public health, general practitioner and hospital services.
1974	National Health Service Act: removed the community health services (maternity, child welfare) from the local authority, establishing the new specialty of community medicine.
1988	Community medicine is renamed public health medicine but remains part of NHS.

Source: First part adapted from Morton 1992

Box 2.1 Effective intersectoral working for health: a case study

City health plans are broad plans drawn up jointly by various agencies in a city to improve the health of its population, as part of their commitment to the WHO Healthy Cities Project. As health is increasingly seen as the responsibility of not just health services, but of all sectors of society, city health plans draw in representatives from key organisations in a city. Costongs and Springett's (1997) paper describes how the plan was drawn up in Liverpool, and explores some of the issues involved in intersectoral working from the participants' perspectives. The study it reports was designed to feed into the process of joint working to aid decision making.

There has been little sociological analysis of joint working for health as yet, although there have been a number of evaluative accounts which identify indicators of effective working, including indicators of process and outcome. In their account of the experience of Liverpool, Caroline Costongs and Jane Springett start from the assumption that indicators of effectiveness will be different for different actors in the process, and that these individual perceptions are a valid subject of research as they will influence collaborative working. They therefore used a methodology based on rapid appraisal techniques, which involve semistructured interviews with key informants from the different types of agency involved, observation of meetings and analysis of reports and meeting minutes. The key organisations involved in Liverpool included the health authority, the city council, community health councils, universities, the trade council and voluntary agencies. An independent Healthy City Unit provided administrative support and coordination for the plan. The plan was drafted by a joint public health team, which had separate task groups working on the specific areas of accidents, heart disease, sexual health, cancer and housing for health.

Participants in the research identified several issues raised by collaboration which may be generalisable outside Liverpool. One was the importance of having senior officers representing their organisations at meetings, who had the authority to make decisions. However, when meetings were chaired by people chosen merely for their seniority, rather than their skills at facilitation and networking, there were problems. The challenge of working with different organisational cultures has been widely reported, and was also reflected in this case study. Here, differences were largely about the concept of health itself, and how it should be promoted, and were particularly evident

between the statutory and voluntary agencies. The relative power
of the city council and the health authority meant that other
organisations had less control over the agenda, and were less
involved in the process.

In summary, the benefits of joint working were that public
health, rather than organisational goals, had a higher priority
and that the plan was jointly owned, which is essential for
effective implementation. The disadvantages were that working
with other organisations is time-consuming, particularly when it is
added as an extra responsibility for staff who may be stretched
already, and that it can be difficult to compromise to reach a
consensus. Costongs and Springett suggest that formal joint
structures are just one element of successful intersectoral working
for health promotion. More attention also needs to be paid to
what they call 'arenas for dialogue': the domains where different
agencies can share each others' experiences and perceptions.

Source: Costongs and Springett 1997

The HFA targets are a direct descendant of the WHO Primary Health Care Conference in Alma Ata in 1977. This initiative
included in its themes the principle of intersectoral collaboration
and community participation (see section on community needs
assessment below for the notorious difficulties associated both with,
and with the lack of, community participation) and resulted in
the creation of a variety of collaborative policy-making bodies,
for example joint committees with members from public health
departments, local authority environmental health and other
officers and community representatives.

Naturally the opportunities for achieving health for all in 15 years,
never mind the little difficulties posed by structural constraints, are
limited. The consequence, then, seems to have been an establishment of joint priorities which would have been on the agenda in
any case – safe (or at least safer) play facilities, a war on dog waste,
HIV/AIDS initiatives, and so on – and to make these the HFA targets.

Subsequent to HFA has been the Ottawa Charter on Health
Promotion (WHO 1986) which will be discussed further in the next
section, and the UK Department of Health *Health of the Nation*
document (1992) which also focuses on the role of health promotion in promoting the public health.

The following extract demonstrates what could be achieved
by collaboration and by a willingness to give a broader brief to
public health, and what happens when this is not backed up by

the necessary political will at both local and national levels, as
Stephen Morton describes:

> My last post was, I believe unique; I was a specialist in Community
> Medicine, based in a large local authority housing department
> (Manchester) with a remit to address health inequalities and
> health problems related to housing. The latter component
> could be subdivided:
> 1 Providing medical advice on the needs of individuals or
> households who were seeking rehousing
> 2 Identifying health needs of homeless people and developing
> strategies to meet these
> 3 Developing housing strategies for client groups with particular
> health needs (ie housing for community care)
> 4 Identifying the effects on health of existing housing stock
> 5 Providing advice on potential effects on health of new housing
> schemes
> 6 Evaluation of new housing schemes.
> Although I wouldn't pretend that it is essential to be a public
> health physician to undertake much of the work which the above
> entails, the areas are all pertinent to public health and offer
> potential for collaboration. Indeed in relation to tasks 1 to 4,
> successful collaboration was achieved; the fact that little progress
> was achieved on tasks 5 and 6 was mainly due to the rapidly
> decreasing amounts approved by central government for the
> Housing Investment Programme (HIP). However an unfortunate
> chain of events successfully eroded the viability of this post.
>
> (Morton 1992: 45–6)

Morton then goes on to describe a series of legislative changes
made by central government that had an impact on the local implementation of policies, such as ratecapping and the restrictions on
reinvesting money made from the sale of council housing; the
Housing Act of 1980 and the Housing and Local Government Act
of 1989 which reduced the role of local government in providing social housing; and the Acheson Report into Public Health
(1988) which recommended physicians should not be involved
in decisions about individuals' priority for rehousing on medical
grounds. The uncertainties over such a marginal post, and indeed
the future of all intersectoral collaborative work, were further
exacerbated by the change to a purchaser/provider system. Indeed
as Morton concluded: 'As far as I am aware, this type of public health
post was not created anywhere else in the UK and, for the reasons
discussed above, it was not refilled in that form in Manchester'
(Morton 1992: 46). Public health has been forever caught between
local government and health, local and centralised organisation,

the short-term and the long-term, the public and the private, the individual and the structural.

The dilemma for public health is that it occupies a 'virtual space': it is constituted by provision, or lack of it, in every other social domain: housing, welfare, employment, law and order, economics, politics. Is it any wonder then that HFA and subsequently Health of the Nation targets were restricted to small-scale achievable, locally based initiatives and that individual education and behaviour change has been the focus of health education and promotion?

Part of the contextualised, holistic approach of the New Public Health is, however, to eschew didactic models of health education and behaviour change and to promote instead models drawn from education theory and community development. The next section looks in more detail at the emergence of 'health promotion' as part of the public health project.

The emergence of new forms of health promotion

From a public health perspective, health education and promotion aim to provide the most effective intervention in order to achieve a health gain (Downer *et al.* 1994). This is often described by the 'upstream/downstream' analogy quoted here from the Preface to Ashton and Seymour (1988):

> *The world is a fast flowing river*
> One of the most common parables told in relation to the New
> Public Health movement is that which equates health workers
> to life-savers standing beside a fast flowing river. Every so often a
> drowning person is swept alongside. The life-saver dives in to the
> rescue, retrieves the 'patient' and resuscitates them. Just as they
> have finished another casualty appears alongside. So busy and
> involved are the life-savers in all of this rescue work that they have
> no time to walk upstream and see why it is that so many people
> are falling in the river. What is necessary, it is argued, is to refocus
> upstream and what is needed generally amongst health workers is
> more 'upstream thinking'. Depending on your perspective you
> may be inclined to conclude that it is people themselves who are
> jumping in and that their sickness is their own fault, that they
> are being seduced or pushed into the river or that all paths lead
> into the river, or that they are the victims of genuine accidents or
> acts of God.
>   (Ashton and Seymour 1988: vii)

Thus, the argument goes, interventions made at the upstream level, that is, in terms of prevention, will be most effective in producing a health gain. To extend the upstream/downstream analogy further, the hospital workers (tertiary care) are forever treating schoolchildren who, when playing on the river bank, fall into the river through the broken fence. The river is polluted as a factory further upstream pumps effluent straight into the river and the children arrive at the hospital suffering from the toxic effects of this. The health intervention can, then, be made at three points, first at the factory level, banning it from putting waste into the river (primary prevention), mending the fence so that children don't fall into the river (secondary prevention), or providing treatment and rehabilitation at the hospital (tertiary prevention). Obviously tertiary prevention will be of only short-term benefit if neither the fence is mended nor the factory effluence stopped. Thus, to be the most effective, health interventions need to be made at each level. In short, in order to promote the health of the public, health policy needs to address the personal, institutional, social, political and economic spheres. (See the discussion of the rise of primary care in Chapter 4.)

Lalonde (1974) popularised the notion of a 'health map' to conceptualise the factors which impact on health. The map has four fields: genetics, individual lifestyle, health services and environment (including social and physical determinants). Health services are, then, only one of a range of factors which have an influence. Others have marginalised the role of biomedical health services even further, arguing that they have minimal impact on the incidence of disease, life expectancy or feelings of health (see, e.g., McKeown 1979; Wilkinson 1996). The field of influences on individual health could be conceptualised as a nested set of factors, with more or less direct influences, as in Figure 2.1.

The determinants of ill health

The question health educators and promoters ask is: where could an effective intervention be made? Clearly there will be structural limits which prohibit much change in health service provision; there is little way of changing biophysical characteristics, although the way services are provided could be addressed (see also the discussion of disability in Chapter 5). Health promotion alone is unlikely to be able to have significant impact on socioeconomic factors. It is easy to see then why efforts to improve the public's health have tended to focus on individual lifestyles and behaviours.

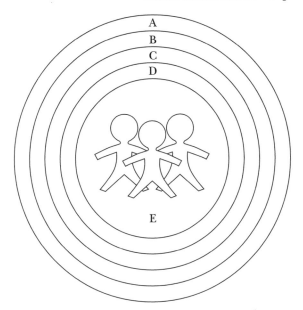

Key: A   Social structural factors: inequality, unemployment etc
     B   Work, housing, environment
     C   Local community, family, culture
     D   Lifestyle choices
     E   Biological factors

Figure 2.1 The determinants of ill health

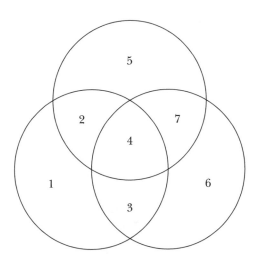

Figure 2.2 A model of health promotion
Source: A Tannahill, in Ashley and Allen 1996: 140

The Ottawa Charter (WHO 1986) promoted the concept of the 'health field', a more complex model of health education and promotion where the differing domains in which health promotion can have an influence are depicted as overlapping fields of prevention, education and protection. These are shown in Figure 2.2, with the following content:

1 Preventive services and facilities, such as school and other screening programmes;
2 Preventive health education, such as the traditional exhortations to adopt healthy lifestyles, found in the main as leaflets, etc.;
3 Preventive health protection, such as legal or fiscal controls and policies and voluntary codes of practice, much of this is derived from old style regulatory public health measures (e.g. fluoridation of water supplies);
4 Health education for preventive health protection; this means lobbying policy makers to make them aware of the importance of, and need for, preventive health education;
5 Positive health education, which aims beyond purely biomedical causes of ill health to encourage 'healthy choices';
6 Positive health protection also aimed at facilitating healthy choices, but at the environmental level; e.g. workplace smoking policies;
7 Health education aimed at positive health protection which aims to raise awareness of the importance of positive health protection amongst policy makers.

Thus the ways in which effective interventions may be made are determined by the type of overlap. It should, however, be borne in mind that this is, after all, only a model. It has a level of detail and complexity which make it almost impossible to translate into practice. The everyday circumstances of front-line staff are more likely determinants of health promotion activity (see Box 5.3 on the administration of waiting lists). Its use is as a tool for analysing policy after it is implemented, not as a model for action.

There have been many models of health promotion, in the main derived from the knowledge – attitude – behaviour model which has been the subject of much criticism. These models work on the assumption that expert knowledge, if effectively imparted to lay people, will change their attitudes (either through fear or through the acceptance of the values) and thus, having undergone this change in attitude, people will alter their behaviour accordingly.

The many critiques point out a number of problems with this type of approach, for example, it fails to acknowledge the structural constraints which limit individual behaviour. This means that failure to change can be held to be the responsibility of the person, leading to a situation which has come to be known as 'blaming the victim'. It also fails to acknowledge that the people targeted may already have important or relevant knowledge (see, e.g., Rodmell and Watt 1986; also discussion of Hilary Graham (1987) in Chapter 3).

The New Public Health eschews the old, didactic models of health education as ineffective, and promotes instead participatory techniques in which people are invited to work at their own pace and to prioritise and contextualise the information given. The aim of this kind of approach is often to 'empower' the community addressed to take action, whether this be individual or collective, social or political (Tones 1986).

How this appears to form part of a broader social transformation can be seen from the case study in Box 2.2 which compares health promotion policy in Britain and Sweden.

Box 2.2 Public health and health promotion as part of a broader social transformation

Gustaffson and Nettleton compare the policy and philosophy of public health and health promotion in England and Sweden. They outline the recent increase in emphasis on health promotion as a strategy for increasing the public health (WHO, HFA etc.) and then summarise the implementation of these strategies in Sweden and England. A number of differences are apparent; for example, Sweden has vague overall aims ('equality of health status') but clear objectives and means to achieve them (improving health of disadvantaged groups via a range of programmes and legislative reforms). England in contrast has clearer aims (improving further the span of healthy life) but not only are objectives and means not distinguished, but the stated means are, the authors judge, 'impressively vague' (p. 10), for example, 'education of the population'. Nevertheless, a move towards the ideas and values of the 'New Public Health' is apparent in both.

There are, as might be expected, clear policy differences. In Sweden, health is seen as rooted in material circumstances, particularly in environmental and occupational hazards, and far less emphasis is placed on individual lifestyle changes, which are viewed as a consequence of social circumstances. In England health is seen as the product of an individual's 'free choice' based on adequate knowledge. Indeed, Sweden's policies are derived from a collectivist and England's from an individualist perspective and it is these historical antecedents which account for their differences.

What, however, interests the authors here are the similarities between the two approaches. Five major similarities are identified: the shift from acute care to prevention ('a move upstream'), a change in policy emphasis from a 'sick' service to a 'health' service; an increase in the surveillance, assessment and monitoring of healthy people; 'health' becoming defined as social rather than merely biological, a positive concept rather than the absence of disease; and finally, the commitment to public participation in health services and the personal responsibility of the individual. Why is it that two states so ideologically and politically different have both produced such similar policy initiatives, that is, national strategies for prevention based on health promotion?

The answer is that this is part of a broader social transformation, one that confirms the social dimension of health and one that requires the monitoring and surveillance of individuals; that is, public health departments now have to find out not only how many, but also who does what and why. The reasons for the emergence of the 'New Public Health', they suggest, might depend on whether it is the policy differences or similarities that are analysed. They opt for the latter, concluding that what we are witnessing is the emergence of new forms of government, what Foucault calls the rules for the 'conduct of conduct' (Burchell *et al.* 1991: 2), of which the 'New Public Health' is one.

Source: Gustafsson and Nettleton 1992

Health promotion as a disciplinary technique

As discussed above, public health has emerged as part of a disciplinary society. It has been deemed a perfect example of the new forms of government described by Foucault (cited in Burchell *et al.* 1991: 87–104), Armstrong (1983) and Nettleton (1992), because it constantly surveys a healthy population with the aim of preventing disease, and this is just what happens in practice. Much of the activity of public health departments is the collection of population-based data derived from routine surveillance techniques, for example, school medical and dental services and the notification of diseases. These then form the basis of subsequent preventive strategies. From a public health perspective this is the currently accepted method for achieving health gains for the population/community. These activities do, however, have unintended consequences: the techniques of monitoring and surveillance leading to the 'action' of health promotion are simultaneously a form and a technique of government. Health promotion might be said to have two effects: it is both normative and normalising (Nettleton 1992). The normative aspects of health promotion are the implicit and explicit values and assumptions (i.e. the form of government). Its normalising aspects are monitoring and surveillance (a technique of government). The case study in Box 2.3 illustrates, with a dental example, how these new public health and health promotion discourses produce social behaviours and norms.

Box 2.3 How discourses of public health and health promotion produce social norms

Sarah Nettleton takes as her theoretical starting point Foucault's concept of governmentality. She discusses how the discursive practices surrounding the mouth and teeth are an example of the way political rule is exercised. Having outlined the notion of governmentality and then considered the 'order of power characteristic of liberal democracy' she then considers the discursive practices which construct an aspect of daily domesticity, tooth brushing. It is, she claims, this routinised behaviour which produces the moral discourse that surrounds dentistry and which constitutes it as a form of government.

Based on dental and archival material and qualitative interviews with mothers and dentists, Nettleton suggests that there is a moral discourse which constructs 'the mother' as 'an agent of dentistry' and that this has moved through four categories: the 'natural mother', the 'ignorant mother', the 'responsible mother' and the 'caring mother'.

Initially, the production of 'reliable statistics' was deemed necessary by the BDA in 1892. This was to provide a knowledge of mouths (wisdom) which would enable the production of the routines and practices (diligence) that would lead to the effective management of teeth. This diligence was to be secured through a range of prevention strategies (dental examinations, epidemiological surveys, health education and social research) in three main sites: dental surgery, school and home.

'The natural mother'

Archival material from the early twentieth century shows that with the advent of routine surveillance in schools, the health of mouths and teeth became seen as an important part of general hygiene. This in turn needed continuous activity, both at school and at home. Not only were teeth to be regularly cleaned but certain foods at certain stages were deemed important for the healthy development of babies' and toddlers' teeth and jaws. Mothers, it was felt, were 'naturally' suited to this function.

'The ignorant mother'

Subsequently however, this became problematic as mothers were ignorant of the 'correct' methods of childrearing. If mothers were to carry out this important function then they had to be trained in the correct techniques. The mouth became a mirror of the child's domestic circumstances and with the mother as the creator and controller of that environment it was imperative that she be recruited and educated to ensure the health and well-being of the population. Failure to do this was perceived as apathetic and neglectful on the mothers' part. Dental health education became part of a moral discourse around the concept of motherhood.

'The responsible mother'

Thus in order for the training and education to be truly effective, it had to arouse the desire in mothers to produce healthy children, to make them active participants in creating the health of their child. They had to want to be 'good parents' and actively pursue those actions necessary within the home to achieve this. From the mid-1940s the ability to co-operate with these goals was seen as related not only to the attitude of the mothers but also to their socioeconomic circumstances. Home circumstances, level of education and standard of living were all seen to contribute to the level of dental caries. Thus it became possible to single out some groups as being in more need of training and supervision than others, with for example, home visits.

'The caring mother'

The responsibility accorded to mothers for the dental health of their children has resulted in them also being held to blame for any dental caries that does occur. The women interviewed by Nettleton articulate this as producing feelings of guilt if they do not get their children to form good habits and eat healthy foods. The quality of mothering can be judged, both by the dentist and by other mothers, by the state of a child's teeth. Currently, this 'negative motivation' is seen as ineffective; rather than inducing blame and guilt dentists should be aiming to harness mothers' enthusiasm. They should be listening to and acknowledging their lay knowledge and creating equal partnerships: mothers who care produce children with healthy teeth.

Thus, Nettleton concludes, mothers have been secured as dental agents and the production of a moral discourse around dentistry has acted to enrol them in the effective practice of government, the production of a healthy population.

Source: Nettleton 1991

Health promotion might then be seen as the 'propaganda' wing of public health, the outrider putting public health policy into practice. How then are we to reconcile this tension between the good intentions of public health/health promotion and the unintended regulatory consequences? First, it should be made clear that this is a false dichotomy. The two aspects are not separable, the one implies the other. The public health discourse implies that a 'reservoir of disease' is a normal part of the social world, but it must therefore be constantly monitored so as to be controlled and prevented. As previously noted, public health could only have emerged in a disciplinary society. To produce 'better health' (a 'health gain') through (public) health policy necessarily produces social regulation, or government (in the Foucauldian sense). (See also the case study described in Box 3.4.)

This is not necessarily a bad thing; there is always 'social control' in one form or another, whether it be 'sovereign power' with punishment as its visible form or disciplinary power with its more subtle technologies (see also Chapter 4). However, what we go on to consider here are the normative aspects of health promotion, in particular in the form it takes as 'empowering'.

There are two points to be followed up here. First, the notion of empowerment itself and second, the potential of empowering techniques. As mentioned, empowerment has been incorporated into the more radical critical approach to health promotion. The concept, however, requires a little further unravelling. Semantically the notion of empowerment implies the transfer of power from one party to another, from health educator to 'communities', that is, from us to them. It would no doubt be argued by health educators/promoters that this is not what is intended; the meaning is, however, embedded in the language. Leaving semantics aside, there remain unresolved problems with empowerment

as a model. The central question surely is '*empowerment for what?*'.
To quote John Ashton and Howard Seymour:

> Health promotion works through community action. At the heart
> of this process are communities having their own power and
> having control of their own initiatives and activities . . . Health
> promotion supports personal and social development through
> providing information, education for health and helping people
> develop the skills which they need to make healthy choices.
>
> (Ashton and Seymour 1988: 26)

These are laudable intentions, indeed ones which many health
promoters pursue in the course of their daily work. But we should
examine this more closely, look behind the rhetoric. The same
phrase 'making healthy choices' occurs again and again in the literature. But what are these healthy choices and who defined them?

While the socioeconomic constraints on choice may be recognised, the value loading of 'choices' is largely unacknowledged.
Unresolved, and mostly unaddressed, is the problem of the freedom to make the 'wrong' choice. The inherent difficulties and
contradictions of advocating this approach are apparent in Tones'
(1986) paper. Tones acknowledges that self-empowerment must
also embody the spirit of voluntarism, that:

> For those seeking to promote self empowerment, the capacity to
> freely choose is success enough even if an individual should choose
> not to reduce his risk of coronary heart disease or steadfastly
> refuses to participate in political activism to close down a factory
> having a poor safety record.
>
> (Tones 1986: 11)

Here is the core problem. Are we really to believe that health
education/promotion and its disciplinary framework, public health
medicine, will be content to measure its success as 'the capacity to
freely choose'? As noted earlier, educational models of health education do acknowledge social structural constraints on choice but
these constraints are regarded as related to class. Tones argues,
for example, that 'free choice' may be curtailed by socialisation
(for example, the 'culture of poverty') or by social inequality.

It is interesting that no link is made here between 'socialisation'
and 'social inequality'. It seems to be suggested that cultural/
behavioural patterns are somehow separate from the social context
in which they are found. It is also implied that those socialised in
the 'culture of poverty' are inferior to those 'whose socialisation
has provided them with self empowering skills and experiences

[and who] have a much greater degree of genuine choice' (Tones 1986: 8).

This more sophisticated health education which takes social circumstances into account further obscures the value-laden agenda. Self-empowerment, then, is 'really' about making 'middle-class' skills and experiences available to the culturally impoverished (at least in terms of health benefits), working class. There is, after all, such a concept as 'genuine' choice and implicit within this is the assumption that empowered people will, for the most part, make (previously defined) 'healthy choices'. Thus critics of the education model maintain that: 'Any attempt, therefore to educate people to make informed health choices in such [constrained] circumstances is not only ineffective but unethical' (Tones 1986: 8), in that they are offering people something they have no hope of achieving.

'Empowerment' facilitates decision making and opens up the issue of choice, of how it is constructed and how constrained. In the process of allowing the messages of health education/promotion to be 'deconstructed', made relevant to their 'target audience', contextualised and chosen, underlying moralities and values are also made visible. Sex education is a clear example. In general 'sex education' is a euphemism for education to prevent unwanted pregnancies and STDs. The moral agenda is that these are undesirable, 'bad' occurrences. With an 'empowering' perspective it has to be acknowledged that this is only one view and that it has no greater validity than any other. Public health/education must then be committed to supporting other choices or forced to acknowledge that it prioritises its own moral perspective which is articulated as 'the healthy choice'. The presence of this tension in public health education and promotion is, perhaps, a major reason for the lack of any widespread use of 'empowerment' techniques. Albeit recognised as more effective learning techniques, it is thought they might also have the potential to render visible the moral aspects of public health or to facilitate the making of 'unhealthy choices'.

Rational choice

There is a further difficulty. Progressive rhetoric holds there is no 'wrong' choice (see above) yet underlying this is the assumption that once in possession of the information, the clarified values and the decision-making skills, and with sociocultural barriers removed, any rational person could not help but make 'the healthy choice'.

This suggests that a critical appraisal of the discourse of rationality might be in order, and it is the location of public health education and promotion within the discourse which is considered next.

One effect of the reliance on rationality is the implicit consensus that health education/promotion has access to knowledge or information which it must seek to promote amongst the public, either as individuals or as 'communities', as this knowledge could benefit the recipients.

Health education/promotion is then charged with using the most effective methods to achieve this transmission. Indeed the semantic shift from education to promotion is seen as evidence of a progression to more effective techniques (Rodmell and Watt 1986; Tones 1986). Thus, whilst the pursuit of public health goals has taken a number of forms, it remains locked within a rational discourse which, however much it is elaborated, basically assumes that in an ideal world increased knowledge leads to changes in attitude and hence to behaviour change. The task, then, becomes to eliminate obstacles to this, not to question the appropriateness of the discourse.

Thus it seems that public health is bound to be less than effective in its project because it is locked within a form of knowledge, the scientific paradigm, which privileges rationality. The object of public health, the 'population' (and within that specifically targeted segments, e.g. individuals, families, communities) is deemed to act rationally. It is, of course, recognised that there are many obstructions to the smooth flow of rational choice and decision making, but that in an ideal world rationality would be the natural state. It is from within this paradigm that the concept of 'a healthy choice' arises. The healthy choice is the rational choice, the medico-scientific choice, the choice that avoids disease and discomfort as defined within medical science. This focus has failed to acknowledge the shifting nature of rationality and has obscured other discourses.

As we are all aware, rationality is contextual and relative. Teenage pregnancy, for example, is problematised in most industrialised societies and normalised in many other contexts. There is not a single rationality, even within the discourse of health. Graham (1987) makes this case forcefully in her work on smoking amongst mothers of young children (as the discussion of Hilary Graham's work in Chapter 3 illustrates).

As stated, the focus also obscures other discourses. Whilst public health education/promotion is premised on rationality, it takes no account of other discourses which construct social interaction. Central to these would be, for example, risk, pleasure and danger. Currently public health presents the 'healthy choice', based on rational discourse. This is constructed as natural, neutral, objective, scientific. Discourses such as pleasure and danger are constructed not as valid alternatives or indeed as coexisting facets of experience, but as moralities, or rather immoralities. The healthy choice of public health thereby conceals its own morality by harnessing 'healthy' to rational, and this becomes synonymous with the sensible, better, correct, choice. These other discourses might be considered disciplines of resistance (e.g. Bloor and MacIntosh 1990), and of course if public health were to embrace these, it would no longer be public health.

Rationality is a product of a particular philosophical world view, or paradigm. Rational choices depend on the very modern phenomenon of risk assessment. Risk assessment and the whole business of insurance, that is, the notion that one can insure against the effects of misfortune (Ewald 1991; Simon 1988), is only possible in an age of statistics, and the use of 'statistics' as an analytical tool is only possible in an era of routine classification, monitoring and surveillance (see Chapters 1 and 6). Thus, risk assessment, and therefore risk itself is produced by the shift from sovereign to disciplinary power.

Risk and health promotion

Contemporary health promotion is based on models of risk assessment. This section will explore this concept of risk and illustrate how sociology has contributed to our understanding of the implications of the 'risk society'. Over the last 15 years there has been an explosion of studies examining risk assessment, and a new, thriving subdiscipline of risk management and assessment has emerged (Adams 1995; Douglas 1986).

In his influential book *Risk Society*, the German sociologist Ulrich Beck (1992) suggested that it is the distribution of risks through which modern industrialised society is divided. New social movements are not formed along traditional class or gender lines but emerge to 'react to the increasing risks and the growing risk consciousness and risk conflicts' (Beck 1992: 90). When Beck discusses 'risk', he refers not to abstract calculations of benefits and dangers, but to concrete misfortunes with everyday implications for the health of the whole population: radioactivity, children with chronic breathing problems caused by sulphur dioxin emissions, poisoned foodstuffs. All societies have had to face danger: what distinguishes 'risk' in late modernity is, for Beck, both the global implications of the risks we face (pollution does not just affect those in the factory, it affects the entire food chain and could potentially destroy the planet) and the 'reflexive' role of science and technology in their generation. We can no longer look to the rationality of scientific progress for the solutions to technical problems, because those problems are themselves the result of scientific progress: science and its critics compete for rational legitimacy. This is illustrated well in the domain of health, where newspaper reports of medical interventions are now as likely to be critical as admiring.

The crisis of legitimacy, and the contestation of accounts of risk, have a further implication for health. Risk assessment has been 'privatised' (O'Malley 1992), in that it has become the responsibility of each of us individually to assess the risks we face and manage them appropriately. A nice illustration of this lies in the *BMA Guide to Living with Risk* (BMA 1990), a publication which attempts to collate the 'objective' statistics on the risks of various activities for lay people. Even with this wealth of scientific knowledge about potential risks, the authors of the BMA guide are careful to note that they cannot give advice: 'It is not possible to make choices for people' (BMA 1990: xviii). People must instead make their own choices, but from a vast array of possible risks, which must be quantified, understood and balanced. Rather than reducing anxiety, knowledge of risks potentially increases it. There are, note the authors, 'few things that are certain in this uncertain and complex world' (BMA 1990: xv).

One thing that is certain is that all are potentially 'at risk'. Robert Castel (1991), discussing how a discourse of risk has fundamentally changed the practice and theory of psychiatry in the late twentieth century, talks of a shift from 'dangerousness', which resided in an individual, to 'risk', which resides in a population. Risks are abstract factors which predispose sections of the population to particular health problems. They are potentially infinite: the growing sophistication of computerised statistics means that ever more subtle sets of risk factors can be deduced. As Castel puts it, they include:

> Not just those dangers that lie hidden away inside the subject, consequences of his or her weakness of will, irrational desires or

unpredictable liberty but also the exogenous dangers, the exterior hazards and temptations from which the subject has not yet learnt to defend himself or herself, alcohol, bad eating habits, road accidents, various kinds of negligence and pollution, meteorological hazards etc.

(Castel 1991: 289)

Prevention can thus be directed at a multitude of levels, and requires constant vigilance: risks must be monitored, and the population surveyed for them.

The sociology of health has also been concerned with how these discourses of risk impact on people's own perceptions of their health and health behaviours in various arenas, such as heart disease (Davison *et al.* 1991), young people's beliefs about AIDS (Warwick *et al.* 1988), adolescents' risk-taking behaviour (Plant and Plant 1993), accidents (Roberts *et al.* 1993; Green 1997) and childhood immunisations (Rogers and Pilgrim 1995).

The example in Box 2.4 looks at the competing discourses of 'morality', 'trust', 'risk' or 'fate' in the way dental patients speak about their management of risk in relation to dentists and HIV.

Box 2.4 The impact of personal risk assessment on health behaviour

This study is based on the qualitative analysis of the nonstructured responses to a street survey eliciting people's attitudes towards the issues raised by the media response to the supposed risk of HIV in dental practice (Allen *et al.* 1992). The 'superficial' findings, that is, those based on responses to a structured questionnaire were that the public had a fairly liberal attitude to HIV-related issues. For example over half the sample thought that an HIV positive dentist should be allowed to go on working and that patients would be prepared to disclose their own HIV status. Most people said they would be prepared to be treated by a dentist known or 'suspected' to be HIV positive. However, analysis of the 'supporting' remarks proved interesting as they articulated attitudes and opinions located in other discourses.

The author suggests that these differences are a result of the operation of two levels of discourse, what Cornwell (1984) calls public and private accounts. Whereas the public account is an expression of the 'socially acceptable' viewpoint, coupled with a desire not to appear foolish, the private account is drawn from alternative discourses which articulate such lay concepts as 'morality', 'trust' and 'responsibility'.

Analysis of these comments suggested four main themes. First, a predominance of references to 'taking the proper precautions' and 'being clean' in relation to being treated by HIV positive dentists. This appeared to have a kind of ritual function; allowing the 'patient' to demonstrate a 'rational response' and was clearly problematic for those who made qualifying remarks like: 'I would like to say yes but it has to be no'. Secondly, respondents typically referred to hygiene, sterility and cleanliness and this became elided with the qualities of the dentists themselves, for example: 'He is a particularly nice dentist, everything is covered up'. It was also important that a dentist was 'trustworthy' and this appeared to be a function of personal knowledge. As both Balint (1957) and Cornwell (1984) note, a good doctor is one known to the person for a long time. Thus the concept of trust conveyed here, and the assessment of risk, was based on the moral judgement of the patient rather than on 'rational evidence'.

Fourth, dentists were construed also as having a professional responsibility, a duty, to their patients. This is a consequence of their role as expert. In all areas of care patients must trust that the dentist is acting in the patients' best interests. In this construction, risks to the respondent personally are deemed best assessed by the professional. This was generally regarded as a reciprocal obligation. Dentists have a right to know their patients' HIV status and disclosure is the moral responsibility of the patient.

Thus the public's response to the media hysteria regarding HIV and dentistry appeared to derive from their perception of their relationship with, and the personal qualities of, their own dentist. Thorogood concludes that 'trust' and 'responsibility' are the counterparts of 'risk'. These ways of thinking should not be dismissed as ignorance or anachronistic but as central to contemporary individual behaviour and decision making. Whilst rational discourses can allow the calculation of risk at a population level, they do not address the assessment of an individual's *personal* risk, for which the consequences of miscalculation are high. Decision making at an individual level can only be based on 'feelings' located in other, antirational, discourse such as morality, responsibility and trust. The implication for dental practice is that it is at this level that the public need reassurance.

Source: Thorogood 1995

Finally, this chapter will consider the dilemmas and debates surrounding that critical activity of public health departments, needs assessment.

Community needs assessment

Since the reorganisation of the NHS into purchasers and providers in 1991, public health has found itself back in a central policy-making role. After all, how will purchasers know what to purchase without good local epidemiology on which to base their assessment? Having an in-built health promotion aspect is often also an essential part of any purchaser's brief. Departments of public health are there to provide the epidemiological research and their health promotion agencies to provide consultancy as to what to include in the brief and then to include it in its own tender. This arrangement looks set to continue, albeit in a modified form. Although the new Labour government are committed to ending the 'Conservative internal market', their manifesto also asserts that 'The planning and provision of care are necessary and distinct functions and will remain so' (Labour Party 1997: 21). Indeed, even before the change in government, 'purchasing' had been transformed into 'commissioning'. Thus public health has found itself drawn in from the cold. No longer is it that wasteland of communicable but unmentionable diseases and no hands-on medicine; rather it is at the vanguard of that currently essential process, community needs assessment.

There are many and lengthy debates around the philosophy and ethics of rationing, which are crucial for determining the process by which resources are allocated. These range from the autocratic to the democratic, with many interpretations of even those conceptual domains (Doyal and Gough 1991; see also discussion in Chapter 3). A great deal of debate centres around the discussion of relativism. Can it be said that there are objective human needs, which pertain to all humans in all circumstances? Or are needs always relative, that is, contingent upon their historical, social and cultural context? Indeed, what is 'need' and can it be distinguished conceptually from 'want', and if so how, and is this universal or relative? Suffice it to say here that at a common-sense level it is accepted that 'health' is a human right and that the provision of health care must be sufficient to meet that need although exactly what is entailed by these concepts of 'health', 'rights', 'provision' and 'need' are the source of much political (both in the general and the specific policy-making sense) dispute.

How then can public health departments go about the task of assessing need? Whose need is going to be taken into account? One useful model of need is Bradshaw's (1972) taxonomy. This is an arbitrary division of 'need' into four basic types, each of which broadly represents the interests of differing sections of the 'health community'. These are: normative need (which is that defined as required for 'normal functioning' by the experts), expressed need (which is the level of use made of the services provided), felt need (which is the perceived need of potential users) and comparative need (which is the difference in needs between groups).

How might these different types of need be measured? (See Chapter 6 for a fuller discussion of the differing methodological approaches.) Expressed need is measured on a routine basis by service providers who maintain records of the use made of their particular service. These have been notoriously difficult to make sense of. For example, the statistical returns for family planning clinics depended on the clinic receptionists ensuring the accurate completion of the record cards. These were almost always incomplete for a variety of completely expected reasons, not least that the data collection had no immediate or apparent relevance to the job of the receptionist. Another example is that of recent increases attendance at genito-urinary medicine clinics; it seems that this is more likely to be a result of the decrease in stigma rather than an increase in need.

Also popular are the epidemiological surveys which are the bread and butter work of public health departments. These measure normative need, that is, the level of 'health' agreed as 'normal', or within the normal range, by the experts. This research determines both the incidence and the prevalence of any particular condition or set of circumstances and it is from this data that local service plans are produced (at least in part). It is from these surveys that indices of treatment need are derived, for example the Index of Orthodontic Treatment Need (IOTN).

Until very recently this has been the sole criterion of need taken into account when funding decisions have been made, giving public health departments a key role in determining resource allocation. As Doyal notes: 'The fairness of decisions about which areas of treatment get what will be a function of the accuracy of the epidemiological evaluation of the relative occurrence of need related to each area' (1993: 52).

However, the building in of health promotion targets to all contracts since the purchaser/provider split has brought different dimensions of need into the frame. As health promotion has shifted into the 'client-centred', 'empowerment' model of effecting health gain, needs assessment has come to mean eliciting the view of either actual or potential service users, that is, the felt need of the general public. This, as might be expected, is fraught with practical and ethical difficulties. Exactly who do you ask? This is a problem of sampling and there are a number of ways of defining a sample, which depend on the aim of the research. Do you, for example, wish to elicit the felt need of the population who are HIV positive in order to provide more appropriate services for this group or do you wish to address the needs of the whole population of whom HIV positive individuals will form a part? This is the difference between providing *targeted* and *general* services and the sampling frame will be different for each (see Chapter 6).

Whole population sampling also presumes that the whole population are potential service users, whereas there may be sections of the population who would rarely, if ever, use the service, for example, young men and general practice, lesbians and gay men and family planning services, and general dental services and those with no teeth.

Nevertheless, whatever lengths are pursued to assess need in all its varied forms, in practice need is often met or rather not met, implicitly. Rationing of health care takes place where the totality of need cannot be met at any given moment in time. In this sense, even given infinite resources, there will always have to be a system for determining who goes first in each treatment queue, as practically not all people could be treated simultaneously. Equally, health need can be met by addressing inequalities in the domain of the social, that is, housing, welfare, education, politics. The relative advantages and disadvantages of the implicit and explicit systems for the planning and prioritisation of health care services will be discussed in the next chapter.

Exercises

Exercise 1

1 List all the 'unhealthy behaviours' you have.
2 Now list all the reasons why.

You may have come up with things such as: pleasure, convenience, habit, cost, religion/beliefs, peer values. The task of health promotion is to change these behaviours, to make normative judgements about which behaviours are acceptable (that is, healthy).

3   Why do you think 'health' is not always regarded as the most important part of life? You have listed competing discourses above. These show how what is important will depend on the individual's 'framework of priorities'.

Exercise 2

1   Make a visit to a local GP surgery, dentist's surgery or health centre and analyse the images used in the health promotion literature in terms of race, class, gender, disability and sexuality.

2   Note not only the images represented but the manner in which they are used, for example, is this a positive or a negative image?

3   Whose values are implicit in health education and promotion?

To what extent do the materials produced as health promotion reinforce stereotypical views of women, of ethnic groups, of appearance and body size, of able bodied and disabled people, of middle-class and working-class people (where middle-class values are privileged)?

Exercise 3

1   Collect as many examples as you can from newspapers and television of sponsorship by food, drink and tobacco companies.

What image are the companies seeking for their product (including a 'healthy image', for example the London marathon sponsored by Flora)?

2   How might the following impact on any government-sponsored health promotion programmes:

   • Corporate interests in sugar, tobacco, alcohol sponsorship, advertising, party political support;
   • International trade in, for example, sugar, tobacco, beef?

3   How might a government health promotion programme consider countering the environmental causes of ill health?

For example, some researchers claim that 80 per cent of all cancers are environmental (Doyal 1979: 61).

What effect might environmental sources of ill health have on the effectiveness of current health promotion strategies?

Further reading

Lupton, D. (1995) *The Imperative of Health: Public Health and the Regulated Body*, London: Sage.

This is an accessible book which takes a Foucauldian approach to the discourses of public health and health promotion. Lupton traces the history of modern public health, and situates its practices within debates on issues such as sexuality, risk, the role of advertising and the body.

Bunton, R., Nettleton, S and Burrows, R. (1995) *The Sociology of Health Promotion: Critical Analyses of Consumption, Lifestyle and Risk*, London: Routledge.

The authors in this collection analyse health promotion from a number of critical perspectives, including sociological, feminist and antiracist approaches. Case studies focus on passive smoking, dentistry, accidents, ageing and consumption.

Chapter 3

Equity in health and health care

Summary: Equity is a key goal of many health policy interventions, although there is much debate about how to define and measure it. Maintaining equity in resource distribution involves making decisions about priorities. In this chapter explicit and implicit models of decision making are compared. We then examine some of the research on inequalities in both outcomes and process in health care, and demonstrate how sociological research has contributed to the policy agenda and our understanding of how structural inequalities such as those of social class or ethnicity are reproduced in the health care arena. For health policy to be equitable, it needs to address a wider arena than health service provision.

Introduction

In evaluating the 'success' of health policy, there are a number of criteria that could be used. One is effectiveness, the extent to which health policies deliver services which do reduce disease or improve health. A second is efficiency, the extent to which this is done in the most cost-effective way. In this chapter, we examine a third criterion, equity, which has been central to NHS policy.

When the NHS was set up in 1948, Aneurin Bevan held equity to be a primary goal. The aim of the new health service would, he said, be to 'universalise the best'. The extent to which it has achieved this aim of divorcing the provision of health care from the ability to pay for it is, then, a legitimate question for policy analysts. How can resources be allocated to health care in a manner that is 'fair' as well as efficient and effective? Unfortunately, there is little agreement about what a 'fair' distribution of resources looks like.

What is equity?

If there are not enough kidneys for transplant for all who need them, who gets priority? If some members of the population are in poorer health because of socioeconomic circumstances, or their own behaviour, should the health service offer extra resources to help them? If people choose to live in remote rural areas, should they be provided with expensive domiciliary dental services in order that their travel costs are not a barrier to equitable access? Answers to these questions about how to achieve an equitable distribution of health care resources will depend on beliefs about individual choice, the proper role of the welfare state, and the ability of the health care services to produce 'health' as an outcome. It should be clear that 'equity' is a contested concept, and the definition chosen will reflect political and ethical values.

There are a number of ways in which 'fairness' could be measured, and they produce rather different results. The economist Julian Le Grand (1991) demonstrates how different conceptions of equity have different implications for policy goals. Equity could mean, for instance, equity of outcome, given that increasing 'health' is presumably a major goal of health services. Here, health policies could be seen as equitable if they produced the same amount of 'health' (in terms of, say, life expectancy or risk of chronic illness) for all groups in the population. Clearly, though, such a conception is rather limited without other information about health needs and other influences on health outside the health services, such as risk-taking behaviour. So a more common measure of equity in health policy is the conception of 'equal treatment for equal need', the idea that resources ought to be distributed only by reference to health care needs. Even leaving for a moment the question of defining what needs might be (this is discussed below), the conception of equal treatment for equal need still poses some ethical problems, argues Le Grand. Should 'just deserts' also influence distribution? He uses the example of a drunk driver who knocks down a pedestrian as an example: if both were equally in medical need of an intensive care bed, and only one bed was available, many people would argue that the pedestrian was the more deserving, in terms of equity (Le Grand 1991: 105), although if the 'equal treatment for equal need' criterion was applied systematically, then the equitable outcome would be either neither were treated, or the decision was made randomly. Furthermore, if we accept 'just deserts' as a criterion when resources are very scarce, why should they not contribute in situations where resources are less scarce, such as reducing health care provision for those who choose to smoke? Distributing health care along such criteria would soon become unwieldy and prone to considerable ethical debate. Another way of conceptualising equity is equity of access: that all members of the population should have the same chances of receiving treatment, whatever their income, geographical location or position in society.

Sociologists have also a long tradition of interest in social inequality. Much social theory and research seeks to understand how divisions in society are reproduced, and what effects economic or other divisions have on outcomes such as health status. There has, then, been a large contribution from sociology in understanding inequalities in health and of producing policy-relevant research in this area.

This chapter starts with a discussion about how recent health policy in Britain has addressed the problem of 'equity' in resource allocation. The second section looks at equity in terms of outcome: the differences in health status that have been observed between different groups within Britain's population. The third examines the process of care: what actually happens to patients as they encounter the health care system. Again, research suggests that experiences of the process of care are systematically related to social position. There is a great deal of sociological research which contributes to our understanding of how health policy both reproduces social inequalities and can potentially help ameliorate them.

Equity and resource allocation

The dilemmas of rationing

As outlined in the introduction to this chapter, resource allocation and priority setting in health care are fundamental aspects of the making of health policy. How should health care resources be allocated and delivered? Given that resources are finite and that demand has to be prioritised, the basis for making these decisions raises moral and ethical questions. A short exercise at the end of this chapter has been included to illustrate some of these dilemmas. Whilst this is an artificial exercise and you may have come up with some creative solutions, the fundamental problem is a real one. What criteria should be used when prioritising health care provision?

Clearly funding levels and government policy have a major effect on the delivery of health care and, whilst no government wants to admit to the rationing of essential health care, in effect whenever need outweighs provision, rationing is taking place. In Britain this has generally taken the form of 'waiting lists': 'Rationing in the NHS has traditionally taken the form of capped budgets and manifests itself publicly in the form of waiting lists' (Rees Jones 1992: 14). Reducing waiting lists then became a political goal in itself, a means of demonstrating action was being taken, whilst in reality the same resources were simply being shuffled round. Thus the government call for action on waiting lists in 1986 (see Box 5.3) meant that in practice quick and simple operations were prioritised over more time-consuming complex ones.

As this example demonstrates, criteria for this decision making can be either implicit (the first-come, first-served waiting list) or explicit (the reduction of waiting lists by doing the simple procedures first). Both are founded on competing philosophical grounds; implicit systems are founded on the principle of individual justice (all claims are of equal value) and explicit systems are founded on utilitarian principles (the greatest good for the greatest number). Both have advantages and disadvantages, and these will be examined in the following sections.

Implicit systems

Up until the recent NHS reforms, doctors in the UK have successfully concealed their rationing behind the discreet cloak of 'clinical freedom'. Consultants were free to treat their patients in whatever way they deemed was in the patient's best interests. This led to an implicit rationing which benefited those with access to care, but disadvantaged those excluded. It also benefited those with acute and life-threatening illnesses over those with chronic and disabling conditions.

An implicit system operates by default and is based on comparative rates of survival following (clinical) interventions. This, however, ignores both quality of life and treatments which are not primarily concerned with life or death issues. As a consequence, dramatic cases are elevated. This produces a situation where cost-minimising accountants are pitched against benefit-maximising clinicians. The allocation of resources is then about who shouts loudest, what Ham (1981) calls 'planning by decibels'. This is also known as 'shroud waving'.

The case of the Halton septuplets provides a very good example of this. In 1987 septuplets, born as a result of fertility treatment, occupied the entire special care baby unit in a Liverpool hospital. Despite several weeks of extremely expensive interventions, none of the babies survived. Whilst it would have been ethically impossible to deny these babies treatment, their monopolisation of the specialist services effectively had this effect on other, less well-publicised, cases. An explicit 'rationing' system would have allowed these treatment decisions to be made on the basis of previously agreed criteria.

The Griffiths' 1984 reform of the health service made an attempt to remedy this by introducing a management tier into the NHS. Where previously clinicians had overall responsibility for hospital administration, the new-style NHS managers were of equal rank to clinicians and employed solely to plan and deliver the most efficient service. This was seen as a triumph of managerialism and intended to limit clinical freedom; however the doctors still had effective autonomy as they had the sole right to admit and discharge.

One consequence of this early attempt to move towards a more explicit system of 'rationing' was the necessity for evaluating treatments and interventions. This was made even more apparent with the 1990 NHS reforms that created the purchaser/provider split. How could contracts be tendered if the treatments and interventions were not costed? This had the knock-on effect of making clinicians justify their use of more costly or complex procedures over other, simpler but seemingly equally effective ones. Thus unquestioned clinical autonomy began to shift in favour of evidence-based medicine, and clinically defined need in favour of explicit resource allocation systems.

It is clear therefore that implicit rationing systems are based on implicit value systems, but how then might these values be regulated? One method is to produce externally agreed criteria for interventions, that is, an explicit decision-making system.

Explicit systems: the advantages

There are a number of models of explicit rationing systems in practice. One famous example of an explicit system of rationing in the USA is what has become known as the 'Oregon experiment'. Faced with budgetary constraints in the Medicaid programme, and criticism of the apparently arbitrary way in which decisions to allocate resources had been made in the past (Dixon and Welch 1991), the Oregon Health Services Commission drew up a list of 700 treatments in 17 treatment categories and, in consultation with the general public, ranked them in order of priority. This system avoided excluding some population groups altogether and instead excluded by treatment group. This was welcomed as a 'scientific' and 'technical' solution to the problem of scarcity (Rees Jones 1992: 12).

Currently, in the UK, many health authorities ration services such as (the highly effective) tattoo removal or breast augmentation whilst many unevaluated or ineffective services continue to be offered, which has more to do with social judgements than rationing based on effectiveness (Pollock 1993). However, the purchaser/provider split in the NHS (and the ensuing obligation for needs assessment), along with the Patient's Charter (ensuring right of access to certain standards of treatment), require Health Service providers to make explicit their decisions concerning resource allocation. For example, they would have to justify rationing by age through the quite arbitrary age cut-off in many coronary care and intensive care units when this is the group most affected and the treatment is effective (Pollock 1993).

One method developed to facilitate explicit decision making is the Quality Adjusted Life Year, or QALY (Williams 1985). The model on which QALYs operate requires the ethical assumption that one year of healthy life expectancy is of equal value to everybody and that being dead is equally bad for everybody (Williams 1987). QALYs are scored on four levels of disability and distress. This matrix is then rated by a sample population and aggregated to give a community value to the quality of life associated with the varied states of health. A profile is created for the time after medical intervention and then the cost is added.

The benefit of this system is that of introducing individual preferences in such a way as to allow them to be used to assess rationally the benefits of alternative treatments. The cost-effectiveness of differing treatments can be calculated and this adds the voice of a

constituency wider than the medical profession in making decisions about resource allocation.

Resource allocation and priority setting are political matters and
therefore the public should be involved, for when responsibility is
not clearly located the rationale of choice is not questioned. In
the UK, where equal access is based on clinical need, an 'Oregon'
style system of consultation could combine technical measures
of benefits with a list of social preferences for rationing, which
would amount to kind of public regulatory system for the internal
market.

After all, who would envy the clinician who has to explain to
several crippled and housebound elderly women in a lot of pain
that they cannot have hip operations because it has been decided
that a 55-year-old man who gets chest pains when he overexerts
himself should have priority (Williams, quoted in Small 1989: 53)?
The introduction of the QALY system means that priorities are
now out in the open.

Explicit systems: the disadvantages

The clearest example of an explicit, utilitarian system taken to its
logical conclusion is that of the necessary sacrifice of one healthy
person to provide the necessary donor organs for seven people
awaiting organ transplants. This system clearly neglects to take
contemporary cultural values into account. However, to take them
into account is also philosophically problematic, for how can we
know what 'notions of rights and justice underpin these "culturally stable value systems"' (Rees Jones 1992: 14) held by the general public?

Clearly, in a democracy, the public's values should somehow be
reflected in any prioritising or ranking of treatment priorities. But
these values may not be homogenous and may indeed conflict.
While in theory the public consultation that occurs in explicit systems enables the voice of the vulnerable to be heard, in practice
these exercises tend to privilege the articulate and the educated.
Few of those involved with the public consultation in the Oregon
experiment were Medicaid recipients (Dixon and Welch 1991),
and as Rees Jones comments:

> It should not be forgotten that these vulnerable groups found
> it most difficult to participate in the consultation exercise. The

OHSC cannot escape the charge of professional elites consulting
with the middle classes to introduce a public 'values system' for
rationing services to the poor.

(Rees Jones 1992: 13)

Other consequences of explicit rationing are that in asking people what they want, and in measuring outcome, you may create a
demand that had only been latent. Consulting the public risks dis-
turbing professional power, bureaucratic inertia and political in-
difference. As Morgan (1993) notes when discussing focus group
methodology (see Chapter 6), beware of asking people what they
want and then ignoring what they tell you.

A further problem is that explicit systems prioritise effectiveness
and efficiency over other criteria for rationing, such as cost utility
or equity, a strategy which also ignores the current reality that the
cost of most interventions remain unevaluated. In practice this
means that clinicians have to refuse to treat poor risk patients. The
recent example of Child B illustrates well the dilemmas posed by
an explicit rationing system. Jamie Bowen, or 'Child B' as she was
known at the time, was an 11-year-old girl with leukaemia refused
further operations by her local health authority as her prognosis
was poor. This provoked a (media fuelled?) public outcry, particularly as the child herself had a very charismatic personality
and was quoted as saying she was not giving up and was determined to live. Eventually her operation was funded privately by a
benefactor and she lived for a further two years.

Thus, whilst explicit systems such as QALYs are based on the
principle that all lives are equally good and all deaths equally bad,
in practice some people's lives, such as the young, or those providing for a family, are deemed of more worth than others, and
these decisions can only be made in a system which allows for
clinical freedom.

Other problems with QALYs are that they are inherently ageist,
as greater importance is attached to duration of life (life years)
than to life itself and need is equated with the ability to benefit.
They do not distinguish between treatments that are life enhanc-
ing (such as hip replacements) and those that are life saving (such
as kidney dialysis) (Hunter 1993). Also, some interventions which
are highly effective, and may reduce psychological morbidity, such
as cosmetic surgery or tattoo removal, are removed from lists of
treatment options based on social judgements. Thus whilst QALYs
may be a fair system for allocating resources at a population level,

they may have an impact on an individual's civil rights regarding equality of access to health care.

So explicit systems are not necessarily 'better' than implicit ones. Calculating the cost benefit of treatments may try to externalise the internal values and assumptions, but it does not take account of those spin-off benefits or costs of particular decisions that cannot be given a monetary value. Nor can an explicit system allow for those 'irrational' aspects of medicine where good practice works but we do not always know why.

Summary of the arguments for and against implicit and explicit systems

The arguments for and against explicit rationing are well summarised by Mechanic (1995). He also elaborates on other, possibly unintended, consequences of an explicit system. He draws our attention to the US system where the majority of the population are affected by 'utilisation management' decisions made by managed care companies. In this system a service is only approved if it is deemed medically necessary, not by the physician recommending it but by the managed care administrators, and although in practice this decision will be made by a doctor it will be made by a doctor acting as an administrator, employed by the managed care companies. This can potentially create a conflict of interests. As Mechanic says: 'When managed care organisations refuse to authorise a service it remains unclear what obligations doctors have to patients to inform them of disagreements about their care' (Mechanic 1995: 1656).

On the one hand doctors may wish to protect themselves against allegations of malpractice by informing patients, but this may lead patients to query the effectiveness of their doctor in acting on their behalf. As Mechanic concludes:

> Differences of opinion between clinicians and utilisation reviewers will contribute to patient dissatisfaction, hostility and lack of trust. . . . Trust holds the system together in the face of economic and other tensions, and in its absence mechanisms of need control are expensive, burdensome and uncertain.
>
> (Mechanic 1995: 1657, 1659)

This may have consequences for patient satisfaction at many different levels (see Thorogood's case study on HIV and dentistry in Chapter 2). At present most people are willing to accept the authority of a doctor, trusting that the doctor will be acting in the best interests of the patient, and will not be making decisions based on financial criteria. Arguably this relationship will be undermined by making rationing criteria explicit. The NHS purchaser/provider split implies a quasi-explicit system, but in practice the system still relies on clinicians allocating treatments wisely within the 'block contracts' that are purchased, and the potential for conflict apparent in a more explicit system makes it likely that it will remain that way. Again, to quote Mechanic:

> Implicit rationing, despite its imperfections, is more conducive to stable social relations and a lower level of conflict. Explicit rationing is also likely to confront government and the political process with unrelenting agitation for budget increases.
>
> (Mechanic 1995: 1658)

A final problem Mechanic notes about explicit rationing systems is that they inevitably give preference to some who care less about treatment than others who are excluded. That is, it takes no account of the different meanings differing interventions hold for each individual. This has implications for the kind of research methods used when attempting to ascertain levels of need (see section on focus groups in Chapter 6).

Currently, most NHS treatments remain free at the point of delivery. Some of the exceptions, such as dental services, are discussed in Chapter 4. However, as funding is allocated on a regional basis there are differences in service provision in differing areas. The previously mentioned examples of both 'Child B' (excluded by an explicit rationing system) and the Halton septuplets (excluding others as the consequence of clinical freedom) might have had very different outcomes if they had taken place in each other's health authority areas. That you might get treatment if you live in one area and not if you live in another hardly seems equitable. One possible solution might be to restrict rationing to within treatment areas rather than between them.

The moral and ethical dilemmas raised by a health service with finite resources are enormous. It is clear that we need a system for prioritising health care. However, it is far from clear what that system should be. The differences between explicit and implicit systems of rationing are summarised in Table 3.1.

Table 3.1 A summary of the differences between explicit and implicit decision-making systems

	Explicit Systems	Implicit systems
Mechanism	QALYS	Expert opinion
Principle	Utilitarian	Principles of justice
Value of lives	All lives equal	Some lives more equal than others
	Quality of life taken into account	'Dramatic' life and death cases elevated (shroud waving)
Rationale	Evidence-based medicine	Clinical freedom
Accountability	Involves public consultation	Unaccountable
Value judgements	Those of 'community'	Those of clinicians

Inequalities and outcome

Health outcomes, such as life expectancy, incidence of disease or self-reported health status, are not randomly distributed throughout the population. There are systematic differences between men and women, between different ethnic groups and between different occupational groups. The place you live also affects your chance of a long and healthy life, independently of these other factors: those living in rural and prosperous areas have the lowest risk of mortality, whereas those in inner city areas have the highest (Charlton 1996). As discussed in Chapter 2, the provision of health services is only one (and probably a small) factor in determining health status, and these inequalities are likely to be the result of the complex web of interacting causes that was illustrated in Figure 2.1. Health policy, to be most effective in terms of equity, should be directed not only at the direct provision of services, but at the point in the social structure where it can make a difference. In this section, the evidence for various explanations of the causes of inequality are examined as a basis for a discussion about possible policy interventions.

The most wide-ranging and best known review of the available research on social class inequalities in health was carried out by the Working Group on Inequalities in Health (Black Report, Townsend and Davidson 1982), which was introduced in Chapter 1.

Table 3.2 The Registrar General's classification of occupations: percentage of male and female economically active adult population in Britain in 1991, in each class

Occupational Class	Examples	Percentage of men	Percentage of women
I Professionals	Doctor, lawyer	7.2	1.9
II Intermediate/ Managerial	Manager, nurse	28.6	28.1
IIIN Skilled nonmanual	Secretary, shop assistant	11.1	38.6
IIIM Skilled manual	Carpenter, bus driver	31.5	7.0
IV Semiskilled	Farm worker, bus conductor	14.6	16.2
V Unskilled	Cleaner, labourer	4.5	7.2
Armed Forces		1.4	>0.1
Inadequately described		1.1	>0.1

Source: Adapted from OPCS 1994, Table 14

Much of the data the group examined used the Registrar General's classification of occupations, which assigns people to social classes in terms of their reported occupation. The percentage of working men and women in each of the classes is shown in Table 3.2.

The Black Report described social class gradients in mortality for most causes of death, with those in the lowest occupational classes and their children experiencing the greatest mortality rates. Similar gradients existed for stillbirths, deaths in infancy, deaths in childhood and in adult life. After 30 years of the NHS, it appeared that the gap between health outcomes for professional workers and unskilled workers had widened. The data they drew on was from the 1970s, but considerable research since then suggests that their findings are still true, and indeed that the gap may be becoming even wider (Davey Smith *et al.* 1990). Between the early 1970s and 1991–3, for instance, mortality dropped by 36 per cent for those in social class I but only by 2 per cent for those in social class V (Drever *et al.* 1996). As Table 3.3 shows, the gradients for some causes of death, including heart disease, lung cancer and suicide, are particularly steep.

Routine surveys, such as the General Household Survey, which questions over 15 thousand households each year, suggest that differences in both morbidity and access to some health care services also persist, although the trends are not as clear cut as they are for mortality. Tables 3.4 and 3.5 show the percentage of adults

Table 3.3 Male mortality rates age 20–64, per 100,000 per year, by social class in England and Wales, 1991–3, for all causes and selected causes

Class	All causes	Ischaemic heart disease	Lung cancer	Suicide
I	282	82	18	13
II	302	93	24	14
IIIN	432	138	35	20
IIIM	496	160	54	21
IV	500	158	53	23
V	816	238	84	46

Source: Adapted from Drever *et al.* 1996

Table 3.4 Dental attendances: percentage of adults who went for regular check-ups, by socioeconomic group

Professionals	65
Employers and managers	63
Intermediate and junior	58
Skilled manual	47
Semiskilled manual	44
Unskilled manual	45

Source: ONS 1997

Table 3.5 Chronic sickness: percentage reporting long-standing illness by sex and socioeconomic group of head of household

	Male	Female
Professionals	24	24
Employers and managers	27	25
Intermediate nonmanual	30	33
Junior nonmanual	29	36
Skilled manual	35	30
Semiskilled manual	36	37
Unskilled manual	35	42

Source: ONS 1997

who have regular dental check-ups by socioeconomic group and chronic sickness prevalence.

General explanations for inequalities

To formulate policy responses to these documented inequalities requires some explanation of how they happen, and to what extent the health service itself can intervene. To what extent, for instance, is the different take-up of preventative dental health service the result of inequities of access such as the number of available NHS dentists, of barriers of cost, or of different cultural values attached to preventative health care? This particular question is explored in more detail in Chapter 4, but if we were to look at other specific areas of unequal access, or unequal outcomes, our answers might be very different. Many researchers have attempted to draw out general explanations, which highlight the major reasons for inequalities in health care outcomes.

The Black Report suggested four kinds of general explanation for these persisting patterns. These were artefact, social selection, cultural/behavioural and materialist. The mechanism that might link health and position in the social hierarchy has been the subject of considerable debate by researchers, and it is possible to find research evidence to back up all of these explanations to some extent.

Artefact explanations

It could be that the apparent relationship between social class and mortality is merely an artefact of the methods used to measure the two concepts, and there is no causal relationship. This explanation relies to some extent on the weaknesses of using occupational groups as an indicator for social class. The Registrar General's Classification of Occupations, which assigns adults to an occupational class in terms of the relative status of the job they do, is often used in health research. It divides the population into six groups, as shown in Table 3.2. It has been criticised as being insensitive to women's employment patterns (as you can see, the distribution of classes among men and women is very different), as lacking any theoretical basis and as being of negligible use over time, given both changes in the classification system and the differing proportions of economically active adults in the various classes. The percentage of men in manual occupational classes has fallen, while those in social classes I and II has risen, with the decline of manufacturing jobs in Britain. The most significant criticism of the Registrar General's classification is that the scale was originally designed to measure differences in mortality rates between groups in the population, so it is hardly surprising that it continues to do so (Jones and Cameron 1984).

However, other research which has used more robust measures of inequality also suggest a similar, or even greater, gradient of mortality risk. The Whitehall studies, for instance, which followed a cohort of 17,000 British civil servants over time, used civil service grade as a measure of inequality and also found a stepwise gradient for risk of coronary heart disease (Marmot *et al.* 1978; Marmot *et al.* 1991).

Social selection explanations

A second possible explanation of inequalities in outcome accepts that there is a causal relationship, but suggests that it is health status which 'causes' social position. Social selection means that the least healthy members of society end up in the lowest social classes, whereas the healthiest move up into higher status positions. If this explanation held true, then there would be little that health policy could do in terms of improving equity in health outcomes. However, although there is some evidence that diseases such as schizophrenia or bronchitis may select for downward social mobility, it is unlikely that health selection could explain the gradients in mortality that exist at all stages in the life cycle. It is difficult to see how social selection could lead to downward social mobility in childhood, for instance, unless there was something about childhood illness that led to fathers taking on jobs lower down the occupational hierarchy as a result. Similarly, differences in mortality outcomes in the postretirement age groups are unlikely to be the result of occupational mobility (Blane *et al.* 1993).

Cultural/behavioural explanations

A third possible explanation offered by the authors of the Black Report was that there was something about the culture or lifestyle of those in the lower social classes which could influence health status. There is evidence, for instance, that people in manual occupations are less likely to eat a healthy diet, and more likely to smoke, as shown in Table 3.6.

If differing lifestyles between the social classes did explain the gradient, then the health policy implications are obvious: that more effort needs to be put into health promotion, and persuading people in social classes IV and V not to indulge in behaviour that damages health.

There are, though, serious drawbacks to the behavioural explanation of health inequalities. The Whitehall studies of civil servants found that even if all behavioural risk factors were taken into account in analysing the different risk of heart disease in different grades, those in the lowest grade were still at 3.6 times the risk of

Table 3.6 Percentage of smokers by social class

Social class	Men	Women
I	13	12
II	22	21
IIIN	25	25
IIIM	32	30
IV	36	34
V	48	33

Source: Colhoun and Prescott-Clarke 1996

those in the highest (Marmot *et al.* 1978). The authors of the study concluded that either there were lifestyle risks yet to be identified (though it is unlikely that any so far unknown risk could account for such a large difference) or that there was something other than individual behaviour that was causing the differential (Marmot *et al.* 1978). Further evidence which undermines the behavioural explanation comes from the Health and Lifestyle Survey, in which a representative sample of 9,000 people in England, Scotland and Wales were asked about their health behaviour and status, and had physiological tests of health status taken (Blaxter 1990). The data suggested that those in the most deprived economic circumstances have *least* to gain in terms of better health status from health-maintaining behaviour such as not smoking, limiting alcohol intake and taking exercise. Mildred Blaxter, in her report of the study, concluded that policy that focused on education about health risks was unlikely to have much impact on the equity of health outcomes as behaviour has little additional impact on social circumstances: 'only in the more favourable social circumstances is there "room" for considerable damage or improvement by the adoption of voluntary health-related habits' (Blaxter 1990: 233).

A further limitation is that even if 'risk factors' are identified as explaining some of the variance between the social classes, this does not get us very far in understanding why risky health behaviours have a class gradient: why should people in occupational class V have smoking rates that are still three times higher than those in occupational class I, despite declining rates of smoking overall?

Materialist explanations

The final possible explanation is that social class influences health status through material mechanisms. There are two ways in which material circumstances can influence health. First are the direct ways, where physical environments damage health or people's material circumstances constrain their ability to maintain their health. Those in the lowest social classes are more likely to live and work in areas where there are environmental risks to health, such as pollution, or hazardous work sites, or poor play facilities for children. They are also less likely to have the financial resources to safeguard their health. 'Healthy' food is often more expensive than unhealthy alternatives. Compare, for instance, the prices of wholemeal and white bread in your local shops.

The second way in which material circumstances can influence health status is indirectly. Here, social structural factors, such as the level of inequality in society, are seen to operate on the health of the population through psychological mechanisms (as yet largely unidentified) which in turn affect physical health. Thus, if you are in a job with poor rewards, in a society where some people are very well off, this might arouse emotional responses which not only make it more likely that you will indulge in risky behaviour (such as smoking or drinking alcohol) but also may directly affect your physical health through their impact on your body's physiological mechanisms.

The authors of the Black Report favoured the materialist explanation, seeing social inequality as the root cause of health inequalities. Work since then has strengthened the case for seeing material factors – particularly indirect ones – as the most useful explanation for health inequalities in industrialised countries. Unpicking the indirect mechanisms by which the social structure can affect the health of groups within it is a methodological challenge, and an area in which much work still needs to be done. However, there is now a considerable amount of evidence that there are indirect material causes of health inequalities, and this has wide-ranging implications for the role of health policy.

Indirect material causes

Richard Wilkinson has been one proponent of social structural explanations of health inequalities in industrialised countries. In reviewing both international data and historical data from Britain, he found that life expectancy tends to be highest when social inequality is less pronounced, and social integration highest (Wilkinson 1989, 1992). The populations of countries which have smaller gaps between the incomes of the richest and poorest, such as Sweden and Norway, enjoy greater life expectancy than those from countries where there are larger gaps, such as the United States and Britain (Wilkinson 1992). Within Britain, historical periods when income differentials have been reduced (such as during the two wars) have been times when mortality rates have gone down. Thus, in countries where incomes are generally sufficient for survival, it is not absolute poverty that affects health, but relative poverty: how deprived you are compared with others in the population. These indirect effects of the social structure on health are perhaps more difficult to comprehend, and also more difficult to address through policy interventions that purely impact on the health sector.

Wilkinson suggests that one key to unravelling the ways in which relative deprivation impacts on health outcomes is to focus on social integration. The notion that social integration affects health is certainly not new – at the beginning of the twentieth century the sociologist Emile Durkheim, in his classic study on *Suicide*, found that rates of suicide were highest in communities where social integration was lowest (Durkheim 1963). Wilkinson cites Putnam *et al.*'s (1993) work on civic society in Italy as evidence that social integration may still impact on health outcome. Putnam used various indicators of social integration including the number of local societies (such as sports associations and charitable groups), turnout in elections and newspaper readership, which might reflect the extent to which members of a society feel part of a larger community. Although not concerned with the impact on health, Putnam does note that the level of civic society in a region did predict infant mortality rates. It is possible that in societies where individual differences in wealth are encouraged, then this kind of community, with its protective effect on its citizens, becomes less important. For Wilkinson, the policy implications of this kind of research are wide-ranging. Improving equity in health outcomes is not, he suggests, an impossible policy goal, but it does involve a multisectoral approach, which includes taxation policies and those affecting the economic climate, as well as attention to the mechanisms which translate relative poverty into poor health outcomes, such as social isolation and psychological stress.

Global explanations, which attempt to explain the general pattern of outcome inequalities, may be of value in thinking about policy at the macro level. The Black Report suggested that, given the strength of evidence for a materialist explanation, the most effective interventions were likely to be those which addressed the economic conditions of the most vulnerable members of society, such as children, through the welfare system. However, more micro level policy interventions may require more detailed information about how particular mechanisms might operate in specific areas of health behaviour and risk, such as smoking, or accident prevention. In Box 3.1, one study of accident risks demonstrates the way in which qualitative studies can illuminate how material factors are likely to contribute to class inequalities in health outcomes, and what the implications might be for policy.

Box 3.1 Some evidence for the material basis of inequalities in childhood accident rates

Background
Accidents are the largest single cause of mortality for children over the age of one, and have one of the steepest social class gradients. Boys in social class five, for instance, have a five times greater risk of dying as a result of an accident than boys in social class one (DHSS 1980). Health promotion has traditionally focused on individual behaviour to reduce the rate of accidents in, for instance, persuading parents to install safety equipment in the home or in teaching children road safety skills.

The study
The study, by Helen Roberts and her co-workers, was based in Corkerhill, a community in Glasgow, which set up an accident prevention group and collaborated with researchers to answer the question 'how do parents keep children safe?'.

Group interviews were held with parents and teenagers who lived in the community and professionals who worked within it. Participants were asked to identify risks children faced in their local environment and the strategies used to reduce them.

Many environmental risks were identified, including electrical sockets with no 'off' switch, busy roads, road works with unattended holes, damp housing, broken glass, broken play equipment and flat roofs accessible to children.

Parents described many strategies utilised to keep their children safe, and they accepted that children's safety was their responsibility. Individual-level behaviours such as cutting down old cots to make fire guards were used, and also community-level interventions, such as campaigns to stop pesticide being used for damp and mouldy houses. When asked how accident prevention could be improved, parents focused on strategies to reduce the number of physical risks in their environments, whereas professionals focused on individual educational strategies.

Implications

Although health promotion aimed at accident prevention has traditionally focused on education, the findings of Roberts and her co-workers (Roberts *et al.* 1992; Roberts *et al.* 1993) suggest that this will have limited impact. Most parents are already well-informed about risk, both in general terms and in terms of the specific hazards presented by their environments. More education risks merely increasing parental anxiety given that there is little that most parents can do to affect environmental hazards.

In addition, the costs of safety equipment (recommended purchases include fireguard, stair gates, cooker guards, safety film for glass, corner protectors and curly kettle flexes) all represent a significant outlay for those on benefits.

More realistic policy interventions in this area would focus on material conditions: on the physical environment children live and play in, or on improving the material resources of their parents. Possible interventions might include regulations for domestic buildings, traffic calming schemes or setting up loan schemes for safety equipment. The most effective approaches to reducing accident rates are likely to be those which involve other agencies, such as local authorities responsible for traffic systems, and involve the communities affected, who are the most knowledgeable about the risks they face.

Sources: Roberts *et al.* 1992; Roberts *et al.* 1993

Understanding why differences in health outcomes persist despite the universal provision of health care is crucial to the development of appropriate policy. Health education can only expect limited success, for instance, if individual behaviour only explains a small proportion of the variation in mortality rates. Furthermore, designing effective health promotion interventions relies on understanding the meaning of risky behaviours, such as smoking, for different groups, rather than merely knowing that they are more likely to smoke. Hilary Graham's work on women and smoking is a good example here (Graham 1987). Graham noted that smoking is associated with disadvantage and caring work among white women: those most likely to smoke are in working-class households and in the most economically deprived areas of the country. She explored the experiences of 57 mothers who were living in poverty, over half of whom were smokers. Graham argues that smoking, for many of these women, was an essential strategy in their task of caring for children in relatively deprived circumstances. Smoking a cigarette marked breaks in a day which was largely taken up with the routines of looking after children and doing housework. It was a way of marking off some 'adult space' psychologically, if not physically, separate from the children. Although women who smoked reported cutting back on their own consumption, even of food and other essentials for themselves, in order to make ends meet financially, the costs of smoking were often seen as the 'one luxury' that would be continued. Again, policy directed merely by education would be unlikely to have a significant impact on smoking rates for women bringing up children in deprived circumstances.

Ethnicity

There is, then, a considerable body of literature which discusses how health policy in Britain has failed to address structural inequalities in terms of social class, and which makes suggestions about how they could be ameliorated. Sociologists have been criticised, though, for ignoring the question of how ethnic differences in health outcomes might be exacerbated by policy, and how the operation of health policy can reproduce racist ideologies (Ahmad 1993; Pearson 1986). Ahmad argues that an equitable health care system would be one in which all members of the population had an equal right to the pre-requisites of health, including decent housing, job opportunities and education, and one in which all could participate as full citizens (Ahmad 1993: 202–3). There is considerable evidence that these conditions do not hold for many of Britain's black and ethnic minority communities, argues Ahmad, and health policy should be understood within the context of arguments about racism and citizenship within the wider society.

There has also been considerable criticism of the researchers and policy makers who, it is claimed, have paid less attention to the structural causes of these differences in health outcomes (such as racism or material disadvantage) than they have to cultural practices, with the emphasis on a 'victim blaming' approach, which seeks explanations in the behaviour of the disadvantaged groups (Donovan 1984; Pearson 1986).

Epidemiologists have perhaps contributed most to our understanding of the differences in health outcomes between different ethnic communities. Ethnic differences in infant mortality rates, for instance, have attracted some attention recently from researchers, as they are a sensitive indicator of health status, and also of access to health services (Balarajan and Raleigh 1990). Andrews and Jewson

(1993) reviewed some of the available statistics, noting that babies of mothers born in Pakistan, the Caribbean, West Africa, the Irish Republic and India all had a higher chance of dying in their first year than those of women born in the UK. Babies born to mothers born in Bangladesh and East Africa had lower mortality rates. When they examined differences at different points in the first year of life, they found different patterns. For postnatal mortality (deaths between one and twelve months old), for instance, only infants born to mothers born in Pakistan had sharply increased rates. Other groups had rates comparable to UK-born mothers, except Bangladeshi and East African mothers, whose babies had lower rates. This finding implied that material differences could only explain some of the difference, given that the Pakistani and Bangladeshi-born mothers share broadly similar economic circumstances. This was also contrary to the expected pattern for the Bangladeshi mothers at least, as they are generally to be found in the lowest socio-economic groups. Clearly no one single, explanatory factor is sufficient to explain the pattern. One problem in developing explanations that are sensitive enough to examine ethnic differences is the limitations of an occu-pational indicator for ethnic communities. The most commonly used Registrar General's classification (see Table 3.2 below) aggregates a number of occupations, and may obscure the fact that in any grouping of occupations, those from ethnic minorities are likely to be in the lower grades, with less job security, and more likely to work shifts.

If secondary analysis of routinely collected statistics cannot provide the whole picture, then qualitative methods may help. The ethnographic study described in Box 3.2 does shed some potential light on the finding that babies of mothers born in Bangladesh are at less risk of dying in the first year of life.

Box 3.2 Using ethnographic work to shed light on infant mortality differences

The problem
The most common cause of death for babies between one and twelve months old in Britain is sudden infant death syndrome (SIDS). Large differences have been noted in the rate of SIDS, both internationally and between different ethnic groups in Britain. Babies born to mothers born in Bangladesh, for instance, seem relatively protected, with rates about half of those born to mothers born in Europe.

Epidemiological studies shed some light on which variables are associated with high mortality from particular causes, but tell us little about how such variables might influence health risks. Qualitative methods can provide some understanding of how lifestyles can put people at risk or, conversely, protect them from particular risks.

The study

Gantley *et al.* (1993) conducted an ethnographic study of 60 mothers of either Bangladeshi or Welsh ethnic origin, living in Cardiff, which involved in-depth interviews. The authors report the broad themes which emerged from these interviews that relate to infant care beliefs and practices.

Results

Typical household patterns differed between the Bangladeshi and Welsh participants. Whereas the Welsh mothers usually lived in nuclear households, the Bangladeshi mothers lived in larger groups, with two or three brothers, their wives and children sharing a house. Many more people took part in childcare in the Bangladeshi households, whereas for the Welsh mothers it was their prime responsibility. The arrival of a new baby usually involved a more dramatic change in lifestyle for the Welsh mothers than it did for the Bangladeshi mothers, who were more likely to live in households with other young children already. Welsh mothers were more likely to emphasise the importance of establishing a routine for bath, meal and bed times, whereas Bangladeshi mothers were flexible in fitting in infant care with other household needs, such as fathers' work outside the home.

Welsh mothers put a greater emphasis on independence for their infants, in getting them used to sleeping in their own rooms, and on taking time away from childcare and housework. They felt it important that babies had quiet to sleep through the day, and that they slept through the night. Bangladeshi infants, and older children, were more likely to sleep in their parents' room, and in the daytime would sleep in the same room as other family members. Infants were placed on the back or side to sleep, to help produce a 'rounded' head.

Implications

Although such ethnographic research cannot prove that childrearing practices have a direct influence on mortality risks, they point to a possible route by which cultural practices impact on biological pathways. It has been suggested that the practice of placing infants on their own to sleep is relatively recent, in terms of human evolution. It is possible that babies sleeping alone lose the 'external sensory stimulation that may stabilise breathing', at a stage of their development when their respiratory systems are not mature. Reporting childcare practices opens up possible avenues for research into factors which contribute to risk of sudden infant death syndrome. Situating these practices within their cultural and social context also provides vital information about the meaning of these practices for mothers.

Source: Gantley *et al*. 1993

Population-level data, as collected in routine statistics, are essential for documenting equity in outcome, but tell us little about the mechanisms by which social inequalities are reproduced as health inequalities, or how policy could usefully address them. They are also problematic for a number of other reasons. First, most sources of information on health in Britain are difficult to link with data on ethnicity. One of the most common indicators used in health research is 'country of origin', simply because this has been the one most often collected. However, given that only about half of Britain's black and ethnic minority population was born outside Britain, this only really captures immigrant health status, which might be very different. The 1991 census was the first which asked for respondents to describe their ethnic origin. About three million people, or 5.5 per cent of the population, described themselves as belonging to an ethnic minority group. The largest communities were those from the Indian subcontinent (India, Pakistan and Bangladesh) and the Caribbean. However, a large proportion of Britain's black and ethnic minority population is of multiethnic origin. This is significant in health terms, as different cultural heritages are likely to have different effects on health beliefs and behaviour, as well as on experiences of being black in Britain. In addition, 'ethnicity' itself is often not the most appropriate indicator. If we are interested in health behaviour, the key variable might be religion. If we are interested in access to health care, it might be language spoken. If we are interested in self-identity, then national identification or self-perceived ethnicity might be important. All these facets of 'ethnicity' overlap, but are rarely identical. In the review of infant mortality rates by Andrews and Jewson (1993) referred to above, for instance, it was noted that infants born to mothers from Bangladesh and Pakistan had different rates of postnatal mortality. These differences would not have been apparent before 1971, when Pakistani and Bangladeshi mothers would have been categorised together.

It is difficult to capture these diverse factors in survey research without ending up with categories which contain too few individuals for any meaningful analysis, although Andrews and Jewson (1993) argue that we should attempt to do so in order to disaggregate the significant variables which may have been aggregated in crude ethnic categories such as 'Asian' or 'Caribbean'. Local ethnographic studies such as the one in Box 3.2 can shed light on these mechanisms for specific causes of death or ill health, and help understand what it is about ethnicity which makes a difference in specific circumstances, and what the most appropriate point of policy intervention might be.

Inequalities in process

The experience of care has long been regarded as an important part of the therapeutic process. First, it can affect outcome. Two examples are studies which demonstrated that good communication in hospital affected length of stay and pain relief needed (Egbert *et al.* 1964) and can improve symptom relief (Fitzpatrick *et al.* 1983). It can also affect access to future health care, in that poor experiences may dissuade patients from returning for further treatment or advice. So although process is not necessarily related to outcome in any straightforward way (see Box 4.3 in Chapter Four), it is a vital aspect of health care delivery. Policies which influence the process of care are important factors when examining how equitable a system is. Qualitative sociology has perhaps most to offer in examining the process of care, and looking at the encounter from the point of view of patients who experience it. One example, discussed in Box 3.3, is an observational study carried out by Isobel Bowler (1993), who described the ways in which racism could impact on the quality of care received by South Asian women at one hospital.

Box 3.3 Racism in the process of care: some evidence from an observational study

The study
Isobel Bowler's study used observation of the maternity department of one hospital and in-depth interviews and 'natural' interviews with staff to examine the care offered to South Asian-descent maternity patients, most of whom were Muslims from Pakistan.

The findings
She found that the midwives held rather stereotypical views
of their South Asian patients. They saw them as 'all the same',
and communications difficulties (none of the midwives spoke
Urdu, and many of the patients spoke little English) meant it
was difficult to form personal relationships. Midwives saw the
mothers as rude and unresponsive. The use of colloquial terms,
such as 'water works', compounded communication difficulties.
   Midwives saw their patients as uncompliant, in that they
did not turn up to clinic appointments, or take prescribed
iron supplements. Staff made the assumption (not always
well-founded) that the women were not interested in family
planning. During labour and postnatally, South Asian women
were perceived as 'making a fuss about nothing', having low
pain thresholds, making noise in labour, and complaining about
minor symptoms postnatally. They were also perceived as lacking
what the midwives thought of as 'normal maternal instinct', for
instance, preferring bottle over breast feeding or not wanting to
hold the baby immediately after birth.
   Some aspects of these stereotypes were the result of lack of
cultural awareness, in that midwives were perhaps unaware that in
Urdu it is uncommon to use words like 'please' and 'thank you'
in the routine ways in which they are used in English.

Implications
Bowler concludes that stereotyping can compromise the care
that South Asian maternity patients receive. Ethnicity becomes
a 'master status', in that it masks differences between women
(such as parity, age, difficulties in labour). Individual needs
are subsumed under assumptions that patients are 'all the same'.
Bowler's fieldwork suggests that aspects of the process of care can
lead to poorer outcomes. For instance, South Asian patients may
be offered inadequate pain relief during labour and staff may
assume that they do not want contraceptive advice.

Source: Bowler 1993

   Studies such as Bowler's raise the question of intervention
to address issues such as racism in health care. How can policy
improve health care delivery, and how can we evaluate health policies in terms of their likely impact on equity? In evaluating policy,
there are a number of outcomes that could be examined. Clearly,
the explicit goals of the policy are crucial, although an almost universal
problem with policy evaluation is that deliberate policy change
is just one factor which might impact on outcome. Sociological

research also has a wider goal, in addressing both desired and undesired policy outcomes, and also engaging in a critical appraisal of policy. Yvette Rocheron's (1988) study of one particular policy intervention – the Asian Mother and Baby Campaign, in Box 3.4, is a good example of an analysis which did this. Although this policy intervention did have some positive outcomes, a critical review also uncovers the unintended negative effects: in this case a reinforcement of racist ideology.

Box 3.4 Critical analysis of health policy: the Asian Mother and Baby Campaign

The Asian Mother and Baby Campaign (AMBC) was a DHSS-sponsored initiative of the mid-1980s which aimed to promote better maternity services for Asian women. Yvette Rocheron examines the medical, social and political contexts of this campaign, arguing that, although the intentions of the policy were to alleviate racism in health care delivery, the result was a reinforcement of racist ideology.

The Campaign consisted of information aimed at Asian families about the importance of antenatal care and a 'link worker' scheme, which employed mutlilingual women to liaise between Asian mothers and health professionals. An initial concern was the policy context of the AMBC, which was an outcome of an earlier, much criticised, DHSS campaign to reduce the incidence of rickets in Asian communities. Here, the interventions had been individualistic, encouraging Asian people to Westernise their diets in order to consume more foods fortified with vitamin D (such as margarine and breakfast cereal) and to expose their skin to sunlight. This approach, and the rejection by the DHSS of a suggestion to fortify chappati flour (eaten by a large majority of those in the communities affected), led to criticism of a 'victim blaming' approach, which advocated personal lifestyle change rather than structural change, and a racist problematisation of Asian culture. Rickets in deprived sections of the postwar white community had been seen as a problem of poverty; in Asian communities it was portrayed as a problem of lifestyle.

The justification for the AMBC was the high levels of perinatal mortality among babies born to Asian-born women. Rocheron notes that perinatal mortality rates are measures of both levels of professional care (those with little access to health care are most at risk) and of health status. The AMBC focused on mothers in terms of their ethnicity, although perinatal mortality rates are also related to social deprivation. The AMBC, like its predecessor, the rickets campaign, identified the problem as one of 'race' rather than one of class.

A second limitation of the campaign, Rocheron argues, was the role of the link worker. These women were employed as interpreters who were seen as assistants to the health professionals, and were managed within the NHS. Had they been independent, they could have fulfilled a more radical role as advocates for the mothers, who could then have challenged medical practice and provided Asian mothers with representation. The training of link workers stressed problems of cross-cultural communication, such as language barriers and differences in naming systems. Built into this, notes Rocheron, is an assumption that racism in health care delivery (such as that described in Box 3.2) is a result of individual prejudice and ignorance, which can be reduced through education and information. Although this may be true to a certain extent, it ignores the level of structural racism within the NHS. Indeed, the first wave of trainers for the campaign were advised not to discuss racism explicitly, in case this alienated NHS professionals, although the issue did reach the agenda in later years of the campaign, as link workers themselves identified racism as a problem in service delivery.

So although the AMBC was a liberal attempt (see Chapter 6) to improve services in the short term for Asian mothers, and undoubtedly had some success in improving communication within health care settings, its limitations were that its approach was piecemeal, locating 'the problem' as ethnicity rather than structural inequalities in health and health care delivery.

Source: Rocheron 1988

Conclusion

The causes of inequalities in the process of health care provision and its outcomes are clearly diverse and interrelated. The challenge for policy makers is to intervene at the level which will have most impact. If structural factors (such as the amount of inequality in a society, or the unemployment rate) do explain most of the inequalities in outcome, then the possibilities for health care interventions appear rather bleak: there is little, perhaps, that this health care system itself can do to ameliorate the systematic effects of social inequality, and even less that individual health care professionals can do. However, we have argued throughout this book that the health policy arena covers rather more than health care services. Tackling inequalities requires far more integration between different sectors, including those which impact on employment and welfare policies, and those which have an impact on social integration.

Exercise

You have a budget of £2,500. How would you prioritise the following 'cases'? This exercise is best done as a group discussion. When you have finished, identify the different sets of values members of the group used to make their decisions.

1 A woman aged 46, unemployed. Needs an osseointegrated (a replacement tooth which grows into the jawbone) dental implant. She can't have a denture due to her strong gagging reflex and because it interferes with her speech and her enjoyment of food.
Cost £1,300

2 A 72-year-old edentulous (i.e. no teeth) man. Needs a complete set of dentures fitted to increase the range of foods he can eat and to improve his appearance and self-esteem.
Cost £350

3 A group of 10 children aged between six and eight years old. All would benefit from fissure sealants on teeth prone to caries.
Cost £150

4 A vicar in his mid-thirties, widowed with two children, is about to remarry a 28-year-old woman with one child. He wishes to have his vasectomy reversed.
Cost £500

5 A woman in her mid-twenties has a large tattoo on her upper arm which she had done as a teenager. She would like it removed.
Cost £425

6 A 17-year-old college student in a steady relationship has accidentally become pregnant. She has decided she wants a termination.
Cost £500

7 A 42-year-old dentist, tested positive for HIV six years ago, now has early symptoms of AIDS. He would benefit from the new drugs treatment/a home nurse.
Cost £1,250

8 A skilled manual worker aged 48 with two teenage children living at home. He has had one severe heart attack and needs a coronary bypass operation.
Cost £1,200

9   A woman in her twenties with three small children. She has one kidney and is on constant dialysis. She needs a replacement kidney.
Cost £1,800

10   A newborn baby is in the special care baby unit with a hole in her heart. Her parents are university lecturers aged 38 and 45; she is their only child.
Cost £1,500

Further reading

Blane, D., Brunner, E. and Wilkinson, R. (eds) (1996) *Health and Social Organisation*, London: Routledge.

Takes a structural approach to inequalities, with chapters from leading researchers on how various levels of social organisation (the family, the community, work and levels of inequality) impact on health outcomes.

Wilkinson, R. (1996) *Unhealthy Societies*, London: Routledge.

Detailed examination of the evidence for relative deprivation as the key determinant of health inequalities in developed societies. This is a readable book, with an international and multidisciplinary focus, taking in anthropological and other literatures to shed light on epidemiological patterns.

Ahmad, W.I.U. (ed.) (1993) *'Race' and Health in Contemporary Britain*, Buckingham: Open University Press.

Overview chapters on ethnicity and health policy, including equal opportunities in the health service, and chapters focusing on current health issues.

Kilner J.F. (1990) *Who Lives? Who Dies? Ethical Criteria in Patient Selection*, New Haven, CT: Yale University Press.

A thorough account of the possible principles that could inform 'patient selection' or prioritisation in health care. Most of the examples are from the USA, but the general issues are, argues Kilner, similar in all health care systems where demand exceeds supply. He considers social, medical and personal criteria as the basis for selection, and proposes his own ethical patient selection criteria.

Chapter 4

Primary care

Summary: Primary care provision has received increasing attention since the late 1980s, culminating in calls for a 'primary care-led NHS'. This chapter outlines recent primary care policy and looks at how sociology has contributed to our understanding of debates about the organisation and delivery of general medical and dental practice. Research on the history of the health centre provides the context for understanding recent policy shifts such as expanding primary care teams and the role of primary care in commissioning. The relationship between patient and professional has attracted considerable attention, and this is one area where sociological research has had some impact. Finally, primary care is used as an illustration to test arguments that health care is becoming 'privatised' to some extent in Britain, with a consideration of the role of charges in dentistry.

What is primary health care?

Primary health care is the first level of contact a prospective patient has with the formal health care system. Within the NHS, most primary health care is provided by general practitioners (GPs), general dental practitioners (GDPs), ophthalmologists and community pharmacists. Patients have direct access to primary health care, unlike other sectors of care where a referral from a health professional is usually needed. Beyond this minimal definition, there are often more idealistic claims made for primary care. In 1972, for instance, the Royal College of General Practitioners defined the role of the GP as someone who 'provides personal, primary and continuing medical care to individuals and families and [whose] diagnoses will be composed in physical, psychological and social terms' (RCGP 1972: 1).

For the Royal College of General Practitioners, the GP is more than a medical generalist. He or she also, ideally, has a more holistic role in patient welfare. For patients, too, the role of the GP may be broader than that of front line health care. GPs legitimise absence from work by issuing certificates, have a role in assessing disability and incapacity for work for benefit entitlements and may be the first port of call for a whole range of social and emotional problems. More recently, the GP's role has also been expanded into areas previously the remit of public health, such as assessing needs and commissioning secondary and community services for patients.

Primary care has also attracted international interest. The World Health Organisation (WHO), in 1978, prioritised primary care as the route to improve health for all. At the Alma Ata conference on primary health care they defined primary care as 'essential health care based on practical, scientifically sound and socially acceptable methods and technology made universally acceptable to individuals and their families' (WHO 1978: 3). For the WHO, primary care included not just medical services, but also education, basic sanitation and preventative measures. Appropriate provision of such care was, the conference declaration noted, a fundamental human right which required the co-operation of other agencies and international social and economic development. Thus health care and social justice were, for the WHO, intertwined. Adequate primary care relied on the participation of local communities and had to be provided in a way which was relevant to local conditions and needs.

Primary care provision in Britain

Since the inception of the NHS, specialist hospital and generalist primary care services have been sharply divided. Primary care meets the majority of health care needs in the formal health care sector: it has been estimated that about 90 per cent of health needs are met by general practice (Glennerster *et al.* 1994). In theory, everyone in Britain is entitled to register with a GP, who undertakes to provide an average of 2,000 patients with primary care and with emergency cover 24 hours a day, seven days a week (often through the employment of deputies to cover 'out of hours' night time and weekend calls). In practice, it is estimated that around 97 per cent of the population are registered with a GP. Although this appears to be good coverage, those that find it most difficult to register may be those in greatest need of health care services. One such group are those without a fixed address. Teresa Hinton's (1994) research discussed in Box 4.1 illustrates the problems that homeless people can experience in finding a GP who will take them on as permanent patients.

Box 4.1 Is there universal access to general practice? Some evidence of discrimination

The problem
Anecdotal and survey evidence suggested that some groups in the population, such as the homeless and recently arrived refugees, were having difficulty registering with a general practitioner. However, it is difficult to assess whether this is a result of discrimination against individuals from these groups, as they are merely told by the surgery that 'the list is full'.

The study
To test whether local GP practices did discriminate against the homeless and refugees, Health Action for Homeless People carried out an investigation using three actors who were asked to play:

- a male Londoner with an unkempt appearance, living on the streets;
- a Kurdish man with little English, moving between squats and friends' houses;
- a white, middle-class woman living in squats with friends.

These actors attempted to register as permanent patients at a range of 30 surgeries in the London Borough of Hackney.

The findings
The actors faced a variety of responses from the surgeries they visited, including the offer of permanent registration, temporary registration, immediate treatment only or refusal to register. The negative reactions encountered meant that considerable debriefing was needed for the actors, who often felt 'shocked, rejected and angry' at the treatment they received. In general,

trying to register with a GP was likely to be a time-consuming
process unless the prospective patient started with one of the
few surgeries which would register the homeless. Results from the
study suggested that those in the most extreme housing situations
faced the most prejudice, as the table shows.

	Percentage of visits resulting in:	
	Permanent registration	Refusal to register
Rough sleeper	14	60
Kurdish man	33	50
Middle-class woman	54	24

Implications
Although in principle everyone has the right to register with a
GP, this study suggests that social factors are likely to impact on
access to care, for certain groups in the population at least. Given
that changing the attitudes of practice staff might be a long-term
goal, and one with uncertain ends, one possible solution might
be to provide tailored care for homeless people.

Source: Hinton 1994

GPs have an important 'gatekeeping' function within the NHS:
they control access to secondary services through the referral system. In Britain, there are few hospital services (other than accident and emergency services) which can be accessed directly by
patients without a GP's referral. The boundary between primary
and secondary care is one area which has attracted considerable
interest in recent years, as attempts have been made to provide
more services in the primary care sector.

As the 'front line' of any health care system, primary care is of
vital concern to policy makers as well as patients because of the
extent of its coverage and its importance in controlling access to
expensive acute facilities. However, in Britain policy in primary
care has had a low profile until the 1980s. One reason for this
comparative neglect could be the contractual position of GPs and
general dental practitioners (GDPs) within the NHS. They are not
salaried employees but contractors, with a tradition of professional
independence. They are essentially small independent businesses,
and it has been difficult for policy makers to dictate policy direction

in primary care: they have relied on the goodwill of individual practitioners, rather than any centralised control. For instance, one aspect of the GPs' ability to act as independent contractors that has been of considerable interest to policy makers has been their freedom to prescribe whatever drugs they feel a patient needs, regardless of cost. Clearly, it is difficult to control spending in primary care if it is not possible to control the amount spent on drugs. Drug companies are very aggressive marketers, and for some drugs there are a range of brands available at very different costs, but which may differ little in their medical effects.

In 1985, the Department of Health succeeded in issuing a restrictive list of prescribable drugs, which contained brands which met all clinical needs, but at the lowest cost. This was successfully introduced despite considerable opposition from GPs, who argued that it was an intrusion on their clinical freedom and professional judgement (see the discussion in Chapter 3 on the conflict between individual and communal needs). This example is a good illustration of the growing attempts in the 1980s and 1990s to plan primary care more effectively.

General dental services

The general dental practitioner has very different origins to that of the GP. As Nettleton (1992) discusses, dentistry is rooted in the discourse of public health and GDPs are primarily involved in prevention and surveillance. Nevertheless, despite, or perhaps because of this, hospital dentistry has had a long and difficult relationship with the medical profession negotiating the boundaries to their respective professions.

At the present time there are three branches to the NHS Dental Service: the general dental service, where each general dental practitioner (GDP) maintains a contract with the FHSA (as do nonfundholding GPs) and is remunerated from the NHS via the Dental Practice Board; the hospital dental service which provides specialist treatment and operates as part of a commissioned provider service (e.g. either a district general hospital or a teaching hospital) and with the same staffing structure as hospital medical services (i.e. consultant, registrar, house officer etc.); and the community dental service (CDS), headed by a community dental officer, which provides community-based services for groups who are deemed to have special dental needs, particularly in relation to access; it also has responsibility for oral health promotion and provides the screening service for all school children. The latter two branches are salaried and the CDS is also purchased by health authorities.

Currently, the majority of qualifying dentists undertake a year's compulsory vocational training, during which time they are salaried, and then start practice as a member of the general dental service (GDS). A small proportion of dental graduates go on to work in the NHS in either the hospital service or the community dental service.

The context: recent primary health care policy

In 1987, the DHSS White Paper *Promoting Better Health* set out national policy for primary care. Its broad strategy was one of increasing the level of control over GP services, and improving standards in primary health care. The major aims were:

- to make services more responsive to the needs of the consumer;
- to raise standards of care;
- to promote health and prevent illness;
- to give patients the widest range of choice in obtaining high quality health care services;
- to improve value for money;
- to enable clearer priorities to be set for family practitioner services in relation to the rest of the health service.

Given that much disease is theoretically preventable, *Promoting Better Health* suggested it could be avoided if 'more members of the public took greater responsibility for looking after their own health' (DHSS 1987: 3). The broader implications of this 'individualising' health promotion strategy were discussed in Chapter 2. Given the regular personal contact that primary care professionals have with their patients, they are ideally placed to deliver preventative health care, including screening for disease and offering health maintenance advice.

One indication of the increasing control the Department of Health exercised over primary care was the successful introduction of a new contract for GPs in 1990, despite considerable opposition from the profession. In line with other Conservative reforms of the NHS, the new contract aimed to bring in more consumer choice and a wider role for the health authority to plan services for their populations. In general, GPs were to be more accountable to the Family Health Services Authorities (FHSAs) which managed their service provision. The main changes to the terms and conditions of service for GPs were:

- an expanded role for FHSAs to plan primary care services for their populations;
- FHSAs to monitor the prescribing profiles of their GPs;
- FHSAs had more flexibility to determine how much ancillary staff costs could be reimbursed, and which staff could be employed;
- introduction of a retirement age of 70 for GPs;
- changes in payments, which rewarded GPs for reaching set targets for the percentage of children on their lists immunised and the percentage of women who had cervical smears;
- that practices should issue practice leaflets describing the practice staff and services offered;
- that it should be easier for patients to change GP.

These changes consolidated the trends evident in *Promoting Better Health*: the payments for reaching targets in cervical smears and immunisations were designed to prioritise prevention work, and the changes to arrangements for paying ancillary staff meant that GPs were able to employ other professionals (such as counsellors or physiotherapists) within the practice. Other changes, such as introducing a retirement age and a stronger planning role for the FHSAs, reflected the perceived need to improve a primary care service which was seen as of uneven quality across the country and unresponsive to either patient demand or central planning. The new contract for GPs was swiftly followed by other changes to primary care organisation brought in by the NHS and Community Care Act 1990, which were based on the 1989 White Paper *Working for Patients* (Secretary of State for Health 1989) and were implemented in April 1991.

The 1990 reforms and fundholding

The changes to the organisation of primary care were perhaps the most controversial part of the Conservative government's 1990 health care reforms. The major innovation was the introduction of fundholding for practices with at least 9,000 patients (reduced to

7,000 in 1993, and down to 5,000 in 1996). Practices, or groups of practices, could elect to be responsible for purchasing non-emergency hospital and (from 1992) community services on behalf of their patients. In terms of policy, the intention was that GPs could influence patterns of secondary care provision through the contracts they placed, and also use any savings made to improve their own practice facilities by, for instance, improving the premises or employing other practitioners, such as osteopaths or counsellors. Potentially, fundholding represents a major shift of power between NHS providers (Audit Commission 1996). General practice, traditionally less powerful than the hospital sector in terms of setting the health care agenda, can now influence how and where secondary care is provided, and also influence the division between primary and secondary care. Fundholding GPs are, to some extent, drivers of the new internal market. However, although there is some evidence that fundholding GPs do impact on the quality of hospital services (Glennerster *et al.* 1994), they are only responsible for a relatively small amount of the total NHS budget. In 1992, fundholder contracts accounted for only about 2 per cent of hospital budgets.

The future for fundholding, and primary care generally, is difficult to predict. In 1996, about half of the population of England were covered by fundholding GPs, and other patterns of GP commissioning are emerging. One of the last central policy initiatives before the Conservative government lost office in 1997 was a White Paper, *Primary Care: The Future* (NHSME 1996), which suggested a period of innovation, with various models of primary care provision being set up for evaluation. One already being evaluated was 'total purchasing', in which the fundholding practice, or group of practices, are responsible for purchasing all their patients' health care needs (TP-NET 1997). There is potential here for considerable impact on secondary care provision.

The new Labour government took office in May 1997 with a commitment to the lead role of primary care within the NHS, and specifically to locality commissioning, with a less wholehearted faith in the ability of markets to achieve efficiency and drive down costs. Before examining current issues in primary care policy, it might be useful first to take a broader view, and examine the context of recent changes. This outline of primary care provision in Britain raises a number of issues for policy analysts. An initial one might be accounting for the recent high profile of primary care on the health care agenda.

Why the attention to primary care in the 1980s?

Allsop (1990) argues that there were three factors which contributed to the renewed interest in primary care policy in Britain in the 1980s: changing population and disease profiles, rising costs and a growing awareness of the variable standards of care across the country.

First, as in other Western countries, an increasing proportion of the UK population is elderly (see Table 1.2), and in need of care for chronic conditions. These changes in population structure and disease patterns have led to an increased focus on prevention as an approach to health care (see Chapter 2), which primary care is ideally placed to do. One of the aims of *Promoting Better Health* was 'to shift the emphasis [of the NHS] from an illness service to a health service offering help to prevent disease and disability' (DHSS 1987: 13).

Second, there has been a trend towards higher referral rates to expensive acute sectors services: the so-called 'clinical drift'. However, family health services account for nearly a quarter of all NHS spending, and the DHSS also noted that rising health care costs affected spending within the primary care sector, given the rising costs of treatment and the considerable investment needed to remedy uneven service provision (DHSS 1987).

Third, throughout the 1980s there was a growing public awareness of variable standards of care across the country. The Acheson Report, *Primary Health Care in Inner London* (London Health Planning Consortium 1981), for instance, focused on the apparent problems in London, which has a higher proportion of elderly doctors, and higher proportion of single-handed practices which are less likely to have the facilities of larger practices and health centres. The use of 'single-handed practices' as an indicator for 'poor practice' is one assumption that has been questioned by sociological research (see Box 4.2), but many health authorities continue to see the reduction of the proportion of single-handed GPs as a policy goal.

Focusing on recent policy changes is important, given the contentious nature of many of the reforms introduced. However, changes in any area of society do not happen just as a result of intentions of policy makers at the centre. If we take a slightly longer term view, it is clear that other trends in primary care provision also have a profound influence not only on the ways in which health care is provided, but potentially also on the kinds of medical knowledge that are produced. One such trend is that of the growth of group practices.

Group practice and the health centre

Until the 1950s, the GP surgery was typically an extension of the doctor's house: doctors consulted in a room of a house which was also their domestic residence. Today, the majority of GPs work in groups, and the trend is towards larger numbers of partners (see Table 4.1). David Armstrong (1985) has examined this change, and the implications for medical knowledge. In the 1950s, GPs worked alone, and there was little division between domestic and work space. This lack of differentiation extended to time, in that doctors of the 1950s may have had definite surgery hours, but were probably on call to their patients all day. They were, in short, 'the doctor' to a local community, often reliant on the family for carrying out their role, for instance in dealing with enquiries when they were out on call.

This configuration of time and space disappeared, though, from the 1960s onwards, being gradually replaced by the health centre as the typical site of primary care. The health centre was a completely separate building dedicated to primary care, where the doctor went out to work during defined surgery times and was on call for defined parts of a rota. Increasingly, the on-call rota would be delegated to special deputising services, who would arrange emergency cover for the GPs.

Various policy initiatives have encouraged GPs to join together in groups to practice. In 1965, the Doctor's Charter provided financial incentives for GPs to join group practices, and policy since then has discouraged the single-handed GP. The decline of single-handed GPs is indicative of this shift in the way that primary care is delivered. In 1952, 43 per cent of GPs worked as single-handed

Table 4.1 Percentage of GPs in single-handed and large (6+ doctors) practices in England

	1975	1985	1995
Percentage of single-handed GPs	17.5	12.1	10.5
Percentage of GPs in 6+ doctor practices	8.8	17.8	26.7

Source: Department of Health 1996

practitioners. Now the proportion is under 11 per cent, and an increasing number of GPs work in large practices with six or more partners (see Table 4.1). The GPs who continue to work alone are, in policy terms, a puzzle: why, with all the incentives to join larger practices, do they prefer solo practice? And why might patients choose (if there is a choice) a small practice with fewer of the facilities offered by a large health centre? Box 4.2 summarises one study which suggested some reasons, and their implications for policy.

Box 4.2 Single-handed GPs: an anachronism?

The problem
Much policy analysis in primary care assumes that single-handed practice is dying out as a pattern of provision. Furthermore, a review of research and policy suggested that 'single-handed' provision is used synonymously with 'poor' provision. However, in some areas of Britain, there are still significant numbers of GPs practising alone: in the area of London where this study was carried out, 19 per cent of GPs are single-handed.
  Given the many incentives to group practice, and the negative stereotypes of single-handed practitioners, why do so many doctors survive in small practices?

The study
The aim of the study by Judith Green was to explore the views of single-handed GPs themselves. A random sample of 25 single-handed GPs from the FHSA's list, and a matched (for age and sex) sample of GPs with partners were interviewed about the satisfactions and dissatisfactions of work, their attitudes to the new contract and to their patients.

The findings
Single-handed GPs in this area were more likely to be male, older and to have trained outside the UK. The services they offered also differed in several ways from their colleagues with partners: they were less likely to employ a practice nurse, to work from purpose-built premises or to run health promotion clinics. Although these are the indicators that are often used of 'good practice' in primary care, the qualitative results from the interviews presented a rather different picture.
  The most striking difference between the two groups of doctors was in the 'style' of practice, or in the rhetorics they used to describe their work. First, the single-handed GPs were more likely to find 24-hour responsibility for their patients a source of satisfaction rather than a stress. Whereas those with partners

---

reported that the most stressful part of their job was out-of-hours cover, the single-handed GPs were often reluctant to hand over 'their' practice to other doctors overnight, and preferred the control of complete responsibility. This was made possible, they argued, because of the 'special relationship' they enjoyed with patients. As the sole doctor, they knew their patients better than colleagues with larger practices, and could offer continuity of care. This identification with the patients was reflected in their talk about the local community: many single-handed GPs reported a feeling of 'belonging' to the local community, whereas the GPs with partners were more likely to stress the negative aspects of the locality when talking about the community (such as deprivation, or the high crime rate). The GPs in partnership identified instead with a professional community, which offered social as well as clinical support. The single-handed GPs saw the professional community as a potential source of stress: often conflicts with partners had been the original incentive for taking on a solo practice.

Implications for policy
The majority of single-handed GPs were very satisfied with their status: they did not want to join partnerships, and financial incentives are unlikely to compensate for the loss of individual control they would suffer. Not all professionals are 'team players' and single-handed practice offers an alternative for those who are not. In addition, they pointed to the advantages for patients: single-handed practice can offer many positive aspects of care (such as continuity and personal knowledge) much more effectively than group practice. Effective policy in primary care should support single-handed practice, as attempts to abolish it are likely to be ineffective and perhaps undesirable.

Sources: Green 1993, 1996

Why does it matter how primary care services are organised? One outcome of the larger practice, argued Armstrong (1985), was a profound change in how health and illness were seen. If the individual solo GP treated individual bodies, in the domestic space of the surgery, the new health centres produced a new space between the domestic sphere of the home and that of the hospital. This new space was the 'community', coterminous with the practice population which was the proper object of health intervention. For GPs, said Armstrong (1985: 661), 'Illness no longer struck unexpectedly at an individual body, but haunted an entire population'. Patient records took on a new importance in group practices, now necessary to provide the all-important continuity, but also a physical manifestation of a new interest in patient biographies. The health centre provided a new location for illness, unique to general practice, and in doing so it produced new ways of understanding health and illness. From this perspective, primary care is the natural location of the new preventative approach to health prioritised by policy makers, and discussed in Chapter 2. It is also helpful in understanding the recent interest in a 'primary care-led' NHS.

The primary health care team and the 'primary care-led' NHS

One facet of the rise of the health centre and demise of the solo practitioner in primary care has been the extension of the primary health care team, including various health care professionals and administrative and managerial staff as well as GPs. The number of practice nurses employed has risen steadily over the last 15 years (NHSME 1996), and since the new contract for GPs in 1990 lifted the restrictions on the range of staff who could be directly employed by a GP, there have also been rising numbers of professionals such as counsellors, osteopaths and physiotherapists who have been employed within the practice (see Table 4.2). The trends towards larger practices (see Table 4.1) and the introduction of fundholding have also led to more managers and administrative staff being employed. Many health authorities are actively encouraging teams within general practice, and supporting those practices which are developing the range of services offered (see, e.g., Lambeth, Southwark and Lewisham Health Commission 1995). In dentistry there has been a recent move towards the notion of creating a 'brand identity' for a chain of dental surgeries, rather like some vets or opticians, which would replace the old dentist/

Table 4.2 Increase in nonmedical staff working in primary care, 1984–94

	1984	1994
Practice nurses	1,920	9,100
Practice staff, excluding practice nurses	24,070	42,734

Source: NHSME 1996

patient relationship based on trust and local knowledge, with a 'label' that would represent certain standards and quality, see for example an article on the corporate image and marketing of 'the Whitecross Surgeries' in *Time Out* (Barron 1995).

Although the idea of a primary care 'team', with a range of professional staff providing integrating care for their locality, is not new, it has not been a reality in many primary care settings. The White Paper *Primary Care: The Future* (NHSME 1996) declared a commitment to teamwork in general practice and the dental team, and to establishing pilot projects to explore different skill mixes in dental teams. This follows the publication of the Nuffield Report (1993) into the education and training of personnel auxiliary to dentistry which recommended extending the areas of work of dental hygienists and nurses and introducing new groups of operating personnel. Parallels can of course be drawn with the shifting division of labour between hospital doctors and nurses (see Chapter 5), and the changes are more likely to be viewed as a consequence of the dentists' pursuit of even more complex or technical procedures than of the increasing status of ancillary personnel. There are indications, though, that the expansion of professionals working with the GP will have an impact on the organisation and division of labour within primary care.

As GPs cease to be solo self-employed small business people, and begin to run organisations that employ many staff, with a complex division of labour, they become structurally more powerful within the NHS. An ever-increasing range of services can be provided directly by primary-care centres, and GPs have an increasing influence on the provision of secondary and community services provided in their locality. This shift in status has been supported strategically from the centre. An Executive Letter, EL (94) 79, *Towards a Primary Care Led NHS*, was issued in 1994. Executive letters are one method by which the NHS Management Executive provides guidance to service managers. Many provoke little comment, but this one had considerable impact. In essence, GPs and their teams are seen as having a responsibility not only for providing the majority of primary care and controlling access to secondary services, but also for assessing and making decisions about health care needs and commissioning services. In the context of reduced confidence in the effectiveness of market competition in the health sector, the new focus is likely to be on collaboration. In April 1996, FHSAs merged with the health authorities (formerly responsible for commissioning secondary and community services), forming integrated health authorities responsible for the whole range of services within their districts (see Figure A.2 in the Appendix). Many different relationships between these new authorities and local GPs have developed across the country, from total purchasing, where a consortium of fundholders commission all care for their patients, through standard fundholding and 'multifunds' of fundholding consortia, to systems where representatives of non-fundholding GPs act as advisory committees for their health authority (see TP-NET 1997; Willis 1996).

As GPs become increasingly involved with needs assessment, prioritisation and commissioning, it has been suggested that their role will overlap with that of public health, discussed in Chapter 2 (Littlejohns and Victor 1996: 7). GPs have changed from being orientated towards the health of individual patients to being public health doctors for their locality, or 'community'. In part, the rhetoric of health providers of course creates these 'communities', which are not pre-existing social groups, but geographical localities defined by the catchment areas of the practices within them.

Despite the continuing debate about how much influence primary care teams will have on the health sector overall, what is of most concern to patients is the quality of service they receive within the surgery. In the next section we turn to the impact of policy on the relationships between patient and professional, and how research has influenced this.

Primary care and the patient

One of the aims of British general practice is that there is continuing and personal care from the doctor. Although the study in Box 4.2 suggested that this may be easier to provide in single-handed practice than the more modern arrangement of the health centre, the relationship between doctor and patient remains a key concern in primary care in all practices. For patients, interpersonal aspects of the encounter are often more important than clinical ones, and personal skills are seen as key to good general practice (Williams and Calnan 1991). Nettleton and Harding (1994) looked at complaints about community services, and found that complaints often centred on these skills, as the main reasons for complaints shown in Table 4.3 indicate.

Table 4.3 Reasons for complaints about community services

Inadequate clinical treatment	27%
Practitioner not responding or co-operating	27%
Personal attributes of health professional	25%
Organisation of practice or staff	10%
Financial issues	7%
Mistakes by practitioner	4%
(some complaints included more than one reason)	

Source: Nettleton and Harding 1994

It is not uncommon for patients to judge the professionalism of their GPs in terms of their interpersonal skills. One complainant in Nettleton and Harding's study wrote of her GP: 'his ability to dispense pills is not in question but his manner – abrupt and abrasive – calls into question his ability as a GP' (Nettleton and Harding 1994: 51).

General practitioners have also long been concerned about the quality of the relationships they form with patients. The work of the psychoanalyst Michael Balint (1957), who suggested that doctors should pay attention to the emotional and social aspects of the patient's story as well as the clinical ones, has had a significant impact on many GPs.

The 'relationship' in primary care is, then, of prime importance to both professionals and their clients. It is also an area that has attracted considerable interest from sociologists, who have studied the factors which influence the quality of relationships in health care settings. The example in Box 4.3, from Mary Boulton and her co-workers, is taken from their larger study, the patient–doctor encounter, *Meetings Between Experts* (Tuckett *et al* 1985), in which they argue that in the modern primary care setting the encounter is best seen as one between a professional, who is an expert in biomedicine, and the patient, who is an expert in his or her own illness.

Box 4.3 The impact of social class on communication: separating process and outcome

Background
There is a large literature on communication in medical settings, and on the impact of social factors such as occupational class on that communication. Much of this literature supports the contention that working-class patients get less out of a

consultation with a doctor, either because of the greater 'social distance' between them and the professional, or because they do not share a common language.

Findings
This study looked at 328 audiotapes of consultations between doctors and their patients, and interviewed the patients one week later. The researchers examined the explanations that were given to patients; strategies used by patients (such as requests for further information, requests for clarification and doubting or disagreeing with the doctor); and the time spent on conversation within the consultation.

The findings supported the argument that middle-class patients were more active in the consultation, in that they were more likely to request further information or indicate their own lay diagnosis of the problem. However, when the authors looked at outcomes of the consultation, they found no significant class differences in the patients' interpretation of the doctor's advice or their commitment to it. So although there was an impact of social class on the process of care, this was not translated into a difference in the outcomes of care.

Implications
Boulton and her co-workers suggest that this may be because doctors do not elicit or respond to the lay beliefs of any patients, whatever their social class. Ironically, they suggest, further training of general practitioners to encourage them to take a more 'patient-centred' approach may increase the significance of social class differences in consultation outcomes, as the more active style of these patients would then perhaps lead to increased benefits from the consultation.

Source: Boulton *et al.* 1986

Such research has had some impact on policy in the area of medical and dental training, where issues of communication are now given more priority, particularly perhaps in postgraduate training for GPs. However, the study in Box 4.3 suggests caution in how far a more patient-centred consulting style will change outcomes for patients. Research has also suggested that this is an area where central educational policy (such as that advocated by the Royal College of General Practitioners) might be limited in its impact on the ground. Michael Walker carried out an ethnographic study of a course for GP trainers, who would be responsible for training GPs, in which he examined some of the limitations of socialising professionals to take on a rather different identity to the one established at medical school (Walker 1988). The course he studied used student-centred teaching methods (with an emphasis on group work, a student set agenda and a focus on process) as a route to self-awareness and to encourage students to reassess the role of the general practitioner. This was to be a model of how the student trainers could relate both to the GPs they would be training and to their patients. During the course, in role plays of consultations with patients, doctors were encouraged to hear the patients' agenda and to meet their needs within the consultation. Walker points to some of the barriers to this kind of approach being continued outside the confines of the course itself, despite the students' commitment to the aims of the course. Tiredness, the demands of busy surgeries and the need for control over the consultation meant that using open questions and practising their listening skills was not always, they felt, appropriate. At the end of the course, there was little evidence that the GPs were any more patient-centred in their consultations than they were at the beginning. Here is one example of a body of research which may have had some impact on the relevant policy community (the Royal College of General Practitioners, for instance), but still has limited impact on practice.

Primary care and the hospital: maintaining the boundary

One of the reasons suggested for the renewed interest in Britain in primary care was that of cost. International comparisons suggest that primary care is cheaper than hospital care, and often more acceptable to patients, given that it is more likely to be local, continuous and co-ordinated. So, in part for financial reasons, there have been many attempts to 'shift the boundary' in British health care: that is, to provide an increasing number of services in the community, rather than in the hospital. Some examples are:

- **'Shared care' schemes.** Antenatal care has long been shared between the GP and hospital obstetric department. Since the late 1980s, there have also been schemes which establish shared care for chronic illnesses such as diabetes or asthma, where the hospital and GP or practice nurse collaborate in treating the patient (Morley *et al.* 1991).

- **Provision of services in the surgery.** Some services, such as minor surgery and pregnancy testing, traditionally only available at the hospital, are now being provided in general practice.
- **'Hospital at home'.** This covers a number of different schemes, involving patients remaining at home for specialist care rather than staying as inpatients. Teams caring for patients can be outreach teams from the hospital or community-based teams. A range of health care problems have been covered by hospital at home, including AIDS-related illnesses, management of chemotherapy and early discharge for hip replacement (Haggard 1996).

Apart from supposed cost benefits (although some of these schemes are actually more expensive than the services they replace), moving services closer to the localities in which patients live potentially provides other benefits. They are more accessible and can afford greater continuity of care, and patients do not suffer from the disadvantages of staying on a hospital ward, such as lack of privacy and difficulties of sleeping because of noise.

At one level, this shift may be attractive to GPs if they are provided with sufficient resources to widen the range of services they offer. Until recently, GPs suffered lower status compared to their hospital colleagues. Honigsbaum (1985) suggested that general practice in Britain has been characterised by two models of care, or two competing schools of ideas about what the proper role of the GP should be, which he calls the 'minor surgery school' and the 'prevention school'. These, he argues, are both reactions to the traditional separation in British health care between the primary and the acute sector, in which general practitioners have traditionally had less prestige than their hospital colleagues. Attempts to redress this, and raise the prestige of general practice as a specialty in its own right, have taken two forms. The 'minor surgery' school advocates that GPs take on more technical services, such as stitching up minor lacerations and performing minor surgery in the practice. In this way, their expertise would become more like that of a hospital doctor.

The second approach, the 'prevention school', characterises the doctors who see their primary role as one of preventing disease and promoting health. As the quote from the Royal College at the beginning of this chapter suggests, this is an approach which is very much associated with the RCGP. Unlike the minor surgery school, which seeks to make GPs more like hospital doctors, this approach seeks to delineate a very distinctive role for the GP, with an expertise that is decidedly community-based, and separate from the idea of the doctor as a technical expert.

In practice, then, how far do these approaches characterise how GPs actually see their role on the ground? A study by Michael Calnan (1988) of GPs' attitudes to the roles they valued looked at three dimensions. The one that is of interest here was the first: their relationship to medicine. At one end of the dimension were those with an exclusive commitment to physical medicine, at the other were those with an exclusive commitment to the psychosocial aspects of care. A questionnaire to measure GPs' orientation, for instance, asked how far they agreed with the statements: 'We are so overburdened with social problems we cannot use the medical skills for which we are trained' or 'The treatment of emotional problems is a major part of the GP's work'. Calnan found that the GPs who were most likely to have a social orientation to their role were more likely to be women, to be under 35 and to be members of the Royal College. In practice, the study concluded, there was little consensus among GPs about what their proper role should be. Both the 'clinical' model of care, where GPs see themselves as technical experts, able to perform a wide range of clinical skills, and what one could call the 'holistic' or social model were found.

Individual GPs are probably offering a differing range of services, and have very different perceptions about what it is they should be doing. Studies confirm that GPs differ in the range of services offered (Whitfield and Bucks 1988). This is, of course, predictable and perhaps proper, given that GPs are professionals with autonomy over their practice. However, this clearly limits the ability of policy makers to influence the division between primary and secondary care, and presents a problem for prospective patients trying to 'guess' whether their GP is the appropriate person from whom to seek care for a particular health need. There are also a number of untested assumptions built into attempts to change the boundary. Angela Coulter (1995) examines two of them: that patients find primary care more acceptable, and that primary care is cheaper. Both, she says, are unproven. First, there is evidence that patients' expectations of specialist care are increasing. Second, there is little data to support the view that primary care provision is cheaper. Many services provided by the GP end up as additional services, rather than ones which replace hospital services. Provision of minor surgery in the practice has, for instance, brought more patients forward for treatment, who would otherwise not have been seen. Although this may be desirable in terms of meeting otherwise unmet need, it clearly does not reduce costs. Again, some researchers have questioned the cost-effectiveness of hospital-at-home schemes (Hensher *et al.* 1996).

Privatisation and primary care

The last section of this chapter deals with the debates about privatisation in the context of primary care. Private consultations with general practitioners represent a very small proportion of encounters in British primary care, but other primary care services, such as adult dental services, are charged for on a fee-for-service basis: costs are borne primarily by the individual at the time of need, rather than by the state. There has always been some contribution on a fee-for-service basis by individuals, but the Conservative reforms of the NHS led many commentators to accuse the government of trying to 'privatise' the NHS and abandon the principles of universal, comprehensive and collectivised health care, free at the point of delivery. To what extent were such concerns justified? The answer, of course, depends on what we mean by privatisation. There are many definitions of 'privatisation', but here we will examine two of relevance to primary care – commercialisation and the retreat of the state from the health care arena – in order to assess the arguments.

Commercialisation

First, we could see privatisation as synonymous with commercialisation, or the introduction of market principles in health care. In this light the introduction of the internal market in itself can clearly be seen to be a move towards privatisation, with the establishment of self-governing trusts which have considerable local authority, for instance to depart from nationally agreed wage levels and to borrow money on the markets. Contracting out nonclinical services has a longer history in the NHS, as health authorities have been required since 1983 to put catering, domestic and laundry contracts out to tender. As Johnson (1990: 94) puts it, 'the NHS has been forced to become part of the enterprise culture and to adopt some of the attitudes and practices of the private market'.

Another aspect of commercialisation is the introduction of profit-type motives into health care. Examples might be the various mechanisms put in to reward efficiency, such as GP fundholders being able to use savings from their budgets to improve practice facilities. Various concerns have been raised that these incentives for efficiency might lead to losses in equity. Would GPs 'cream skim' patients, that is, refuse to register those patients who are likely to make expensive demands on their practices, such as those with long-term chronic conditions, or those in deprived economic circumstances? In their study of the implementation of GP fund-holding, Glennerster *et al.* (1994) found no hard evidence of such practices, but said that they remained a theoretical possibility until formulas for paying GPs were adjusted to make 'cream skimming' uneconomic.

The other way in which commercialisation could be seen to be happening is in terms of charges that can be made for certain services, such as prescriptions or spectacles. The introduction and raising of charges for primary care services has been described as 'privatisation by the back door' (Birch 1986). Although charges have never provided a large proportion of NHS revenue, they have tended to be raised by Conservative governments. Dentistry raises 25 per cent of costs through direct charges to patients. The rationale for direct charges is partly that charges deter trivial attendances, in that they introduce an element of self-rationing into publicly provided health care. The other way of looking at this, though, is that they may have a deterrent effect, and that people in need of services may not get them.

How has this affected primary dental services? GDPs are part of the NHS, but, like nonfundholding GPs, they operate as small independent business people. Some GDPs work completely outside the NHS, that is, they see only private fee-paying patients. Some GDPs do only NHS-funded work. For the most part though, GDPs offer a mix of private and NHS care within their practice. This has become increasingly the case since the change to the funding of the Dental Service in 1992. At the present time, children, adults on income support, pregnant women or mothers with a child under one year are entitled to free dental care under the NHS, whilst all other adults are required to pay four-fifths of the cost of treatment. The 1992 changes also altered the system for paying GDPs:

> Remuneration combines two elements, capitation payments and item of service payments. For children, capitation payments

cover routine care (treatment and prevention). Special items
such as endodontic treatment, treating traumatised incisors
and orthodontics attract additional fees. For adults the reverse
is the case: item of service payments continuing to be the main
component of fees and continuing care payments a much smaller
component.

(Gelbier, in Downer *et al.* 1994: 53)

The change in the way dentists are remunerated has had a significant impact on the level of NHS care available in some areas.
Research (Consumers' Association 1992) has shown that access to
NHS dentistry has decreased amongst certain groups, noticeably
fee-paying adults, and this is reflected in the decrease in the
number of NHS registrations amongst those eligible for a contribution to treatment costs. GDPs have become increasingly unwilling to take these people on to their lists, as treatment costs are
fixed centrally and may not reflect the reality of a practice's over-
heads. Thus, although a practice may take NHS patients, in reality
this may be limited:

... a dentist's level of commitment to providing NHS dental care
can vary from treating an occasional patient to a full time service.
Some dentists accept only certain categories of patient or carry out
a limited range of treatment under the NHS, perhaps providing
a mixture of NHS and private dentistry in the same practice.
Examples include: treating all children plus adults exempt from
dental charges under the NHS and fee paying adults privately; or
providing routine care only under the NHS and certain items such
as dentures, crowns and bridges privately. Dentists working in
general practice are self-employed (except for a few salaried
practitioners) and hold in tension the responsibility of being
caring health professionals on the one hand and small
businessmen or women on the other.

(Gelbier, in Downer *et al.* 1994: 47–8)

This remuneration policy, as Gelbier notes, creates a dilemma for
the practitioner. It also creates tensions for the public.

It is well-documented that the two biggest barriers to dental care
are cost and anxiety (Finch *et al.* 1988) and that only approximately
50 per cent of the adult population regularly attend a dentist. The
reasons for this are, of course, many and varied, depending, as in
other aspects of health care, on factors such as the level of service
provision as well as social factors and the model of risk which
underpins people's perception of their oral health care needs. For

many people, oral health care has a very low priority (along with other parts of the body considered marginal, such as feet). This contrasts with the presumed regularity of personal oral health care: tooth brushing and the six-monthly check-up. For some 'dentally anxious' people, adherence to this schedule ensures the continued absence of pain and possibly painful interventions. For most others, whether anxious or not, only the presence of dental pain will trigger a visit to the dentist.

The effect of the system of payment for dental treatment is to exacerbate these contradictions. As the research of Finch *et al.* shows, most people do not regard dental treatment as a high priority and cost as well as anxiety has acted as a prohibitive factor in their uptake of services. Currently, however, it appears that 'cost' is a source of anxiety. There is widespread confusion amongst the general public about the level of dental charges (Finch *et al.* 1988) and the effect of the 1992 changes has been to add to this. Charges for NHS dental treatment are not new; they were introduced in 1950 (the first part of the NHS to depart from Bevan's ideal of a service totally free at the point of need). However, until recently, these charges were perceived as nominal and were not based on a fee-per-item system. The 1992 changes in remuneration for dentists, requiring patients to make a proportionate contribution to the cost of each of the procedures undertaken, have made apparent the true costs of dental treatment and the relative differences in cost between different procedures.

The consequences of these changes in funding on service access and use are complex. Rather than the predicted 'end of NHS dentistry' (as widely reported in the English national press on 7 July 1997) it seems that there are certain areas, particularly some London boroughs, in which it is hard to register with an NHS dentist: 18 per cent of those surveyed by the Consumers' Association had difficulty finding an NHS dentist, compared to 7 per cent nationally (Consumers' Association 1992). Another consequence has been the production of uncertainty over potential charges. It has been suggested that this confusion over charges acts as a barrier to seeking care. According to the *Which?* survey, 17 per cent of the sample had put off their next appointment because their dentist would only see them privately. It is likely that this uncertainty will extend to those who don't know whether or not their dentist will treat them on the NHS, or those who are not registered with a dentist, meaning that surveys such as this may underestimate problems with access.

When charges are not clear or predictable the patient is placed in a difficult position. What if the dentist recommends, or worse, carries out procedures you can ill afford? At what point do you say, as to a garage mechanic, stop, please let me have an estimate before carrying out any repairs? Equally, if a dentist is explicit about the cost of the treatment how can a patient say, no, they prefer to continue with the rotten tooth or whatever than pay for the work suggested. After all, in matters of health, the healthy choice is seen as the rational one (see Chapter 2) and to suggest instead that you would prefer to spend the money on something else would brand you irresponsible in regard to health.

The dentist–patient relationship is that of professional–client; clearly, if the dentist thinks work needs to be done, it is not the place of the patient to question this professional judgement. To do so would undermine the relationship, particularly from the patient's perspective, as it could be tantamount to admitting a lack of judgement in your choice of professional. It might also cause the dentist to react badly to ostensibly having his or her clinical judgement questioned. The fear of potentially being in such an awkward position may act as a deterrent to seeking treatment in anything other than an acute situation (Finch *et al.* 1988).

It has been recommended that dentists display their charges (Finch *et al.* 1988) and this would go part way towards remedying these uncertainties. However, even with this improvement, the final cost of treatment would still remain unclear as interventions cannot, necessarily, be accurately predicted.

It is not just in dentistry that rising commercialisation has had an impact on access. Charges appear to have also had a deterrent effect on access to eye tests. As Table 4.4 shows, the number of eye

Table 4.4 Number of general ophthalmic service eye tests

Year	Number (Thousands)
1988	11,695
1989	12,493
1990	5,280
1991	4,154
1992	4,979
1993	5,528
1994	5,935
1995	6,383

Source: DOH 1996

Table 4.5 Complaints about family health services leading to formal investigations

Year	General medical services	General dental services
1988	1,232	436
1989	1,361	423
1990	1,339	500
1991	1,608	472
1992	1,445	426
1993	1,891	540
1994	1,862	508
1995	1,788	427

Source: DOH 1996

tests carried out in England has dropped dramatically since the introduction of charges. Indeed, eye tests have shifted from being a statutory right to being an individual responsibility; a current advertising campaign urges people to ensure they have regular eye tests 'before it's too late', thus attempting to persuade us to revise our priorities in favour of health checks. This self-surveillance can be interpreted as an extension of disciplinary power.

An increasingly 'commercial' approach to health care has implications beyond those of access. It also potentially affects how professionals feel about their work and how they relate to patients. One outcome of increasing commercialisation of the patient–doctor and patient–dentist relationship in primary care may well be the increasing willingness of patients to complain about the services they receive. As Table 4.5 shows, the trend has been towards increasing numbers of complaints about both GPs and general dental practitioners. Of course, there may be many reasons contributing to this trend, including wider cultural shifts in the trust we have in 'experts' of all kinds, but it is perhaps inevitable that if general practice looks more like a 'business' then patients will be willing to complain if services are not what they expect. However, an alternative reaction is that, given the reduced choice of dental practitioners who offer NHS services, patients may be reluctant to complain in case they are deregistered by their dentist and are unable to find another to take them on (Thorogood 1997a).

The retreat of the state

A second way in which we can think about privatisation is as an outcome of the retreat of the state from providing health care.

From this perspective, privatisation is about the 'decollectivisation' of health care, in which it is seen less as the obligation of the whole community and more as a private responsibility. The state can potentially intervene in health care in a number of ways, the extent of which may vary from state to state. It can:

• *directly provide* health care, by employing health care professionals and providing facilities;
• *subsidise* health care by, for instance, subsidising health insurance, or collectivising the costs of health care through taxation;
• *regulate* health care provided by others, for instance by inspecting hospitals and residential units, by legislating minimum standards for services, or regulating criteria for professional registration and training.

These are very different sorts of activities, and if we are looking at how far the state has retreated from health care provision, our answer might be rather different for each.

In terms of direct provision, the White Paper *Working for Patients* left the state as the major provider of health care, although it did encourage a renewed co-operation between the private and public sectors. In the hospital sector, managers have had to put support services (catering, laundry and domestic) out to tender since 1983. One trend of interest in primary care is the increasing range of 'alternative' or 'complementary' practitioners who provide, in theory, front-line services. Although in practice many patients may visit complementary therapists (such as acupuncturists, Chinese herbalists, aromatherapists, homeopaths or hypnotherapists) as a last resort for problems which are not adequately dealt with by their GP, they do provide an accessible alternative for first contact. It is estimated that one in seven of the British population visit alternative practitioners (Saks 1994). 'Complementary' therapies cover a wide range of health professionals, working in very different systems, and motivations for self-referral to specific practitioners are consequently diverse. One study (Lam and Green 1994), for instance, found that members of the Vietnamese community sometimes used traditional Chinese practitioners rather than negotiate language barriers to the use of NHS GPs, and preferred medicines with instructions in Chinese. Given that very few of these practitioners, or those of other complementary professions, work for the NHS, most consultations and treatments have to be paid for on a fee-for-service basis.

It would be difficult to attribute this growth directly to policy shifts within the NHS. Clearly, this is an area where wider social change, including a questioning of biomedical approaches and perhaps greater tolerance of alternative rationalities, impacts on health behaviour. However, Saks (1994) notes that recent health reforms may widen the provision of alternative practitioners within the NHS, as GPs can employ other therapists to provide primary care for their patients. Given consumer demand for these therapies, and incentives for GPs to respond to consumer demand, numbers working within NHS health centres may increase. Alternatively, biomedically trained professionals may increasingly utilise therapies developed by their 'alternative' colleagues. Speculatively, this is one area where the health reforms may reduce demand for private health care, if this demand can be met within the NHS. It is debatable whether this will result in the higher profile and status or in the medicalising of alternative or complementary therapies; indeed, the answer may lie in the name: will these services remain alternative to biomedicine or simply become complementary? As noted earlier in this chapter 'counselling' is already a commonly featured service in general practice, although what is offered tends to be very short-term (six weeks) rather than the in-depth therapy offered by modern psychotherapists. (For an interesting discussion of psychotherapy from a Foucauldian perspective, see Nikolas Rose's 1990 book *Governing the Soul.*)

If we turn to collectivising the burden of costs for health care, there is certainly evidence that although GP consultations are still free at the point of delivery, patients are having to pay more on a 'fee-for-service' basis for various kinds of primary care, as discussed in the last section.

There has been considerable policy analysis on the provision of private medicine and its implications, but to understand the process fully it is also important to look at the 'demand' side: why might patients choose private medicine when an NHS alternative exists? As most of the private provision in Britain is of secondary care, this has attracted most of the research (see, e.g., Higgins 1988; Calnan *et al.* 1993). However, there are some studies of the attitudes of primary care patients. One study, by Nicki Thorogood, on why black women might choose to pay for primary care, suggests that paying a 'fee for service' might meet the needs of some patients who are in a structurally weak position in obtaining good quality NHS services. See Box 4.4.

Box 4.4 Private primary care: buying some equality

The problem
Research into private medicine has neglected primary care. Little
is known about the motivations of those who use it. Black women
are one group who are more likely to pay for a private
consultation.

The study
In-depth interviews were carried out with 32 women, aged
between 16 and 30 or between 40 and 60, from one London
borough. All the older women were born in the Caribbean and
had moved to Britain in the 1950s and 1960s, and about half of
the younger group had been born in Britain.

Findings
For many of the women interviewed, experiences of 'back
home' (the Caribbean) included using private health care. About
half of the sample had used private health care in Britain, and
many others would consider it if necessary and if they could
afford it. For these women, private health care meant a private
consultation with a general practitioner, not the purchase of
private health insurance. Thus they were not, like Calnan's
(Calnan *et al.* 1993) respondents, buying convenience or
specialist skills. The majority of women supported the NHS, and
politically saw private doctors as a 'necessary evil', to provide a
quality of service which the NHS ought to provide for them
but did not. Private doctors provided a certain set of services
unavailable to them on the NHS: a second opinion, a thorough
examination (which NHS GPs were seen as too rushed to do),
regular check-ups and more time. One, asked to describe who
would use private doctors, said: 'The rich . . . unless you're a
person who, you know, is not rich, but you want to get proper
treatment'. Another participant said of private doctors: 'They are
certainly quicker to examine you and they seem more thorough'.
    What is at issue, suggests Thorogood, is that paying for a
service gives patients a certain amount of power which is not
apparent in their dealings with the NHS. For women who are
black, working-class and live in deprived inner city boroughs, the
NHS provides a service which may be second best, and which
treats them as powerless and vulnerable. Directly paying for
services restructured their relationship to their doctor: from
that of passive and powerless beneficiary to that of active client.
Although critical of the structural reasons for inequalities within

the NHS, the women interviewed, as black, working-class women, could not personally affect changes in the system. Paying for a consultation with a practitioner reliant on personal referrals is a rational way of extending control over their own health care.

Source: Thorogood 1992

Primary care is likely, then, to continue to be the subject of considerable policy debate. There are unresolved questions about how primary care services should be organised, how they are to be funded and what they should consist of. If calls for a 'primary care-led' NHS are successful, the structure of health care provision in Britain could be changed significantly. As the research discussed in this chapter has shown, changes in health care delivery have wide-ranging repercussions. The expansion of GP practices into complex organisations impacts on professional–client relationships and on what medical practice itself consists of. The trend towards commercialisation within primary care impacts on access and potentially on equity. There is much scope for sociological research which explores the changing organisation of primary care and the effects it has.

Exercises

Exercise 1
Collect a range of practice information leaflets from GP and dentists' surgeries and compare the services offered.

Using friends or colleagues as a 'sample', carry out a 'mini-survey' on people's use of primary services.

What 'alternative' therapies do they use?

Are there any barriers to their use?

Exercise 2
Describe some possible implications of the expansion of primary health care for:

• patients,
• health care workers,
• the state.

To what extent may the following occur and what might their effects be on patients, health care workers and the state?:

- health services may become more accessible,
- health services may become more integrated,
- Primary health care workers may have more job satisfaction,
- Primary health care workers may feel under more pressure,
- there may be a change in the site of resistance (see Bloor and McIntosh 1990), as it is perhaps harder to 'resist' (i.e. to refuse) someone you know personally, than to resist a faceless bureaucrat.

Further reading

Jones, R. and Kinmonth, A-L. (1995) *Critical Reading for Primary Care,* Oxford: Oxford University Press.

Shows how various disciplines and methods contribute to research for primary care. Authors of each chapter have been asked to choose a paper reporting research, which is reprinted with their critical commentary on the paper, why they choose it and the broader context. Also has useful advice on doing literature searches in health (for instance, using databases, and critical reading).

Tudor Hart, J. (1988) *A New Kind of Doctor: The General Practitioner's Part in the Health of the Community,* London: Merlin Press.

A personal account of working in the NHS (from the author's experience of being a GP in Wales), how general practice has changed and a radical vision of the contribution general practitioners could make.

Littlejohns, P. and Victor, C. (1996) *Making Sense of a Primary Care Led Health Service,* Oxford: Radcliffe Medical Press.

Chapters on key facets of the move towards a primary care-led NHS, including the role of commissioning, needs assessment, audit and information needs, with some examples of local innovations.

Chapter 5

Health care organisations: management, professionals and their patients

Summary: By the nineteenth century, hospitals had become the dominant site of both medical training and medical treatment. The role of the hospital in the delivery of medical care is, some argue, now in decline, and the hospital itself has become a contested area of policy interest. This chapter examines some of the ways in which institutional context impacts on health care: on medical knowledge and on relationships between professionals and their clients. Sociology has a long tradition of interest in the relationship between bureaucracy and professional power in organisations, and this has contributed to research on the process of hospital management, the division of labour within the hospital and the impact of hospitals on medical knowledge. Nurses, although the largest group of health care providers in hospitals, have been marginalised in terms of policy and research. Criticisms of the hospital, particularly for long-term care, have revived interest in 'community care'.

Introduction

A number of questions about health care organisations exercise many of those responsible for health policy, including the Treasury, the Department of Health, local managers who decide on resource allocation and pressure groups concerned with local services. Hospitals are central to the organisation of modern medicine, but their dominance is being questioned in several respects. One is their declining role in long-term care, for groups such as the mentally ill or the elderly. At the end of this chapter, we will return to this in a consideration of 'community care' as an alternative to institutional care. It is not just the decline in long-term care which has changed the nature of the modern hospital, though. The introduction of general management to the NHS in the 1980s and its consolidation in the 1990s has changed the hospital as an organisation. Moves towards a 'primary care-led NHS', discussed in Chapter 4, have shifted the boundary between the hospital and community, and raised questions about where certain services are best provided. There is, however, still debate about whether there are enough beds in NHS hospitals to provide inpatient care for all those in need, or whether London, for instance, has too many. The distribution of hospital services also causes debate: should services such as cardiac surgery or major trauma be centralised so that they are delivered by the most experienced professionals, with most effective use of expensive resources, or are services best provided locally?

The role of research

Research cannot provide answers to these questions, as they are rooted in value judgements about what the proper criteria are for health care: whether, for instance, it is about providing the most effective service in terms of lives saved or extended, or the most efficient in terms of most benefit for money spent, or the most humane, in terms of perhaps situating services where communities want them (see Chapter 3). One example of plans to centralise services comes from the Calman–Hine report on commissioning cancer services (DOH 1995). This advocated the establishment of cancer centres, which would provide specialist services to populations of up to a third of a million, as well as more generalist cancer care for those within their immediate locality. The rationale for centralising care was that of *effectiveness*: that research demonstrates better outcomes for patients with certain cancers if they are treated by specialists. The report also urged more research to evaluate services provided for patients in terms of their effectiveness. However, effectiveness is not the only criterion that is important for commissioners, providers and patients of health care services. Ahmad (1993), for instance, discusses the losses to equity that an exclusive focus on effectiveness or efficiency might entail:

> Under the [1990] reforms some 'specialist' services will only be provided at regional level. Health reforms are thus likely to exacerbate the current problems of access and equality for

minority ethnic groups.   None of these likely developments offers
much comfort for the ethnic minorities for whom accessibility and
equality may include considerations of language, dietary and other
specific needs in addition to the problems of individual and
institutional racism.

(Ahmad 1993: 206)

If research cannot adjudicate between different values, or criteria,
it can provide some evidence on which to judge the relative merits
of different policies. There is a burgeoning multidisciplinary area
of health services research, which empirically tests some of the
assumptions built into health policy, such as 'the most experienced
professionals provide the most effective health care' or 'the largest
hospitals are the most cost-effective'. Sociological methods, along
with those of other disciplines such as economics, contribute to
these areas of research. In this chapter we will examine some of
these contributions to our understanding of how policy has impacted on hospitals, including studies of how the locus of medical care impacts on the nature of the care delivered, the division
of labour in hospitals, the impact of management and the implementation of strategic policy. The sociology of hospitals is also a
rich field for the sociology of policy, as illustrated here by some
of the work on how management is achieved in hospital settings
and the ideological background of community care. To put this
work in context, we start with accounts of the rise and (heralded)
decline of the hospital as the major locus of medical work.

The rise and decline of the hospital

Although hospitals have existed since the Middle Ages, the institutions we recognise today as the organisational centre of medical
treatment and training emerged in the late eighteenth century. It
has been argued, from a range of theoretical perspectives, that the
emergence of the hospital as the major site of both treating disease
and teaching future doctors had a wide-ranging impact not only
on how health care is delivered, but on what medical knowledge
itself consists of (Ackernecht 1967; Foucault 1976; Jewson 1976).

Foucault's account of the role of the hospital

Michel Foucault (1976), in *The Birth of the Clinic*, looks at the rise
of the Paris hospital in the late eighteenth century, and argues

that the new locus of medical care in the hospital rather than the patient's home enabled a new kind of medical knowledge to be produced. One precondition for this new knowledge was a new understanding of anatomy, and the gradual breaking down of taboos against the dissection of corpses. This brought with it a radical change in the way in which disease and death were conceptualised. In the sixteenth and seventeenth centuries, disease was regarded as an external agent that invaded the body. The new understanding was of disease and death as part of life: disease was part of the organs and functions of the body itself.

Foucault called this new understanding the 'clinical gaze'. This phrase implied a particular way of seeing bodies and the diseases they carried which penetrated them, examining them for the underlying pathology. For Foucault, this new gaze was a facet of a new kind of power, a power that relied on surveillance and inspection. With hospitals now teaching institutions, rather than merely hospices for the poor or infirm, doctors had large numbers of patients to examine, compare and, if they died, dissect. For Foucault, the hospital is just one example of the kinds of institutions which developed in modern secular societies – the school and the prison were others – which were sites at which the state could control the population. They represented a new kind of power, not based on the absolute soverignity of the king, but on a more pervasive and controlling power which acted on individual subjects (see also Chapter 2).

The model of this new kind of power was Bentham's Panoptican, a plan for an ideal prison. In the Panoptican the cells are arranged in a ring around a central tower, from which a guard could potentially see any inmate. Windows from the tower to the cells were shuttered, so the prisoners would never know when they were being observed and therefore had to assume that their behaviour was under constant surveillance and act accordingly. The classic Nightingale hospital ward has elements of this arrangement, with patients arranged so that they are visible from a central nursing station, and their bodies, in night clothes, ever ready to be subjected to the various examinations and inspections of the medical gaze.

Foucault's analysis is at the level of discourse: what it is possible to say and know, and how it is said, and indeed how and what we see when we look. He starts his book *The Birth of the Clinic* with a quote from Pomme, a medical writer from the middle of the nineteenth century, who describes how he cured a hysteric by making her take 'baths for ten or twelve hours a day, for ten whole months'. At the end of this treatment, Pomme saw:

> membranous tissues like pieces of damp parchment . . . peel away with some slight discomfort, and these were passed daily with the urine; the right ureter also peeled away and came out whole in the same way. The oesphagus, the arterial trachea, and the tongue also peeled in due course.

(Foucault 1976: 1)

It is not merely that no modern doctor would treat a patient thus, or indeed even recognise the disease of hysteria, but that a modern doctor would *see* the body, and its constituent parts, in an entirely different way. The new medical 'gaze' which Foucault talks about is not just an act of looking; it also involves the techniques of physical examination, and more significantly, it makes the invisible signs of pathology visible, providing a way of seeing the anatomy of the body in a new way. Thus the anatomy which is mapped in books such as *Gray's Anatomy* (Gray 1962) is not, for Foucault, an unchanging reality, always there but only recently discovered, but rather it is a product of a specific discourse.

Jewson's account of the role of the hospital

Another writer who has looked at the changes in medical knowledge over the same period is Jewson, who takes a more Marxist approach by looking at different stages of medical knowledge in terms of their modes of production: the social factors inherent in the relationship between the client and the provider of that knowledge (Jewson 1976). Jewson discusses 'cosmologies' of medical knowledge, by which he means something similar to Foucault's discourse. A cosmology is a conceptual structure which frames the kinds of things that are known, what questions may be asked and the kinds of answers that are offered. For Jewson, however, these cosmologies are not merely cultural artefacts but are produced within certain economic relationships, and medical knowledge is intricately tied to the kinds of economic relationships which give rise to it.

Before the end of the eighteenth century, argues Jewson, the major mode of production was what he calls bedside medicine. Bedside medicine was not characterised by any one unifying theory, but included diverse schools of thought: there were many conflicting accounts of disease and healing. However, what these different medical theories had in common was their focus on symptoms as experienced by the patient: the manifestations of illness rather than its underlying causes. It was a holistic approach, taking all the factors of a patient's experience into account to find the original cause of the illness. Medicine was essentially person-orientated. The practitioners were fragmented as an occupational group, and their livelihood depended on the goodwill of their patrons, the patients. The status of clinicians was dependent not on their clinical skills, defined by an autonomous profession, but on the status of their patrons.

With the rise of the hospital, says Jewson, this mode of production was replaced by one of hospital medicine, which rested on a new relationship between the sick patient and the practitioners. First, social roles were now prescribed rather than negotiated between individual patrons and practitioners. They were prescribed so that the practitioners had the respect and deference that had been won by organising as a coherent profession. A new object of medical cosmology emerged here: the disease, rather than the sick patient.

Hospital medicine, argues Jewson, made four innovations:

- **Structural nosology:** the idea that diseases could be classified, by either causative agents or parts of body, rather than their effect on the patient.
- **Localised pathology:** the idea that particular organs or systems are diseased, rather than the whole person.
- **Physical examination:** as the key to diagnosis, rather than verbal reports from the patient.
- **Statistical analysis:** the large numbers of patients in one place in the hospital meant that they could be compared.

By the beginning of the nineteenth century, then, medical education had been institutionalised at the hospitals, replacing the theoretical education of Oxford and Cambridge Universities for physicians and the apprenticeships for surgeons that had preceded them. In Britain, this development was consolidated by the 1858 Medical Act which established the General Medical Council which was to regulate the medical profession on behalf of the state, and to oversee medical education. It was this Act that perhaps finally established medicine as a profession, as the council were to keep a register of qualified medical practitioners. It made it illegal for anyone but a registered medical practitioner to call themselves such and joined all recognised healers (formally in different organisations

Table 5.1 Number of beds and consultants in NHS hospitals
in England

	1984	1990/1	1992/3	1994/5
	Number of acute and general beds ('000)			
Available inpatient beds	194	163	153	145
Day cases	875	1,251	1,785	2,439
	Number of hospital consultants			
	13,214	15,520	16,263	17,099

Source: DOH 1996

as surgeons, physicians or apothecaries) on to one register (see
later in this chapter).

For the following century the hospital continued to be the dominant organisation in the delivery of health care. Doctors and nurses
have been trained within the teaching hospitals, and hospital doctors have enjoyed more status than their counterparts in general practice. However, at the end of the twentieth century, the
centrality of hospitals has come under increasing threat. Chapter 4 briefly examined some of the attempts to shift the boundary
between primary and secondary care, and to stop the 'clinical drift'
towards hospital care. There are several indicators for the declining role of the hospital as the defining locus of medical care. One
is the reduced amount of time that inpatients actually spend, on
average, in hospital. As Table 5.1 shows, there has been a gradual
trend towards a reduction in inpatient beds and an increase in
'day case' treatment.

The declining number of beds and length of stay in NHS hospitals presents a problem for medical education, traditionally centred on the 'ward round' in which the consultant visits each of his
or her patients, accompanied by students who are taught by the
bedside (Atkinson 1981). Solutions to this problem have also moved
the focus away from the hospital (Oswald 1989). One London
scheme, for instance, has moved a medical 'firm' (a period of
clinical training) into general practice, where students learn in
the community what was once learnt in the hospital ward (Tucker
1991). There may be many unintended consequences of policies
which shift care and training into the community (see below for a
discussion of the term 'community'), and there has been some

speculation about the likely impacts on relationships between doctors and their patients. Andrea Sanker, in her study of a similar scheme in the United States in Box 5.1, suggests that the institutional environment has a significant effect on the kinds of relationships which develop between professionals and their clients.

Box 5.1 The impact of context on relationships: providing care outside the hospital

This study specifically examined the impact of context on the nature of interaction between doctors and their patients, through a case study of the effect on medical students of treating patients in their own homes.

The medical school Sankar studied requires its students to participate in a Home Care programme: a period during which the student is responsible for three to four seriously ill and housebound patients. Instead of treating these patients in the hospital outpatient clinic, the students visited them in the home.

Sankar notes that the attachment was an unpopular one with the students to start with. When she asked what one student hoped to get out of it, he said, 'Myself, as quickly as possible'. Students were concerned that they would not learn much from a home care attachment, that it would not be intellectually challenging, and they would get frustrated by the limited scope there was for 'curing' medical problems. They had negative attitudes towards caring for people with chronic conditions, preferring to practise medicine which 'made a difference'. As their programme progressed, and the students got to know their patients better, their attitudes changed, and many focused more on the patient's individual needs, social and emotional, as well as medical. Many found that the information patients disclosed as 'social' information, which would not have arisen in the doctor-controlled interview in the hospital clinic, was actually vital in terms of understanding their medical problems. Some students found the whole experience a troubling and difficult one. For some students, it undermined knowledge learned in other parts of their course.

Sankar argues that the context of the encounter – the patient's home rather than the physician's office – crucially affects not only the kind of relationship that emerges between patient and professional, but the kind of knowledge that can be produced. In the patient's home the doctor is on 'their turf' as one put it, and the nature of the relationship is very different to that created in the clinic: the patient has more control over the encounter. Undressing the patient for an examination requires negotiating,

it does not happen automatically; washing hands involves asking
for the sink; leaving may require exchanging personal
information with the patient, rather than just receiving
it, and possibly taking the part of the 'guest' and accepting
refreshments. In sum, the trainee doctors had to relinquish
some of the control they took as unproblematic in the hospital
clinic. The result was that they inevitably treated the patients in a
more holistic way than would have been possible in the clinic, as
they were aware of the impact of illness on everyday home and
family life as well as on the body. For some students, this led to
a reappraisal of their view of medicine generally, and a sense of
nihilism that there was little benefit in medical interventions for
patients with chronic problems. Rather like the client-centred
mode of production identified by Jewson (see discussion above),
Sanker's students had to shift their practice to a more patient-
centred mode, in which the patients set the agenda for their care.

Source: Sankar 1988

However, despite these indications of the declining role of the
hospital as the major provider of many kinds of medical intervention, and the interest in community-based teaching programmes,
hospitals are likely to continue as important sites of training and
care for some time to come. Sociological interest in the hospital
has traditionally centred on questions of organisation, and has
informed much of the debate on these issues.

Understanding hospital organisation

Sociology has had a major part to play in the understanding of
hospital organisation. Hospitals are large, powerful institutions with
a complex division of labour, and sociologists have focused on
questions such as how order is achieved in such settings, and how
certain groups in the occupational structure exert more control
than others over that order. They have also contributed to our
understanding of the impact of the organisation on patients.

The conflict between professional and managerial power

Studies of organisation often take the work of the turn-of-the-
century sociologist Max Weber as their starting point. Weber (1949)

argued that bureaucracy was a particular kind of hierarchy, characterised by a separation of the officials and the posts they occupy. In bureaucratic organisations, there is a hierarchy of offices, to which people are recruited and promoted through merit (indicated, for example, by examination passes) rather than personal influence or heredity. Neither the post nor any of the resources that go with it (such as equipment or payments for services) can be appropriated by the official, as they belong to the office, not to the official who occupies that office. Bureaucratic officials carry out their duties according to predefined rules and protocols.

Weber's model was an 'ideal type', and of course it does not describe exactly how hospitals, or any other institutions, are organised. However, there are aspects of this kind of organisation which are typical of hospitals (and many other institutions of modern society). What is particularly interesting about hospital organisation, though, is that bureaucracy is not the only source of authority. Medical professionals derive their authority from rather different sources, and their lines of accountability are very different from those of managers. As professionals, doctors derive authority from their practice of specialised skills, their theoretical knowledge, their state-legitimated monopoly over practice and their ideology of 'service' to individual patients. An ideology of 'clinical autonomy' means that doctors treat each patient as an individual, and can make decisions about their health care needs without reference to wider questions about resources, priorities or management protocols. Much has been written on medicine as a profession, indeed it is in many ways the archetypal profession, its traits used as benchmarks to judge the professional claims of other occupational groups.

Eliot Freidson, in his classic study of the profession of medicine (Freidson 1970), argued that the status of doctors derived not from a core of specialised knowledge, nor an orientation towards service, but from the strategies that had been used to gain a monopoly over practice. Only the profession itself can determine what constitutes medical work, who is legitimately able to do it and how it can be done. 'Professional autonomy' in practice means that individual doctors in a hospital have an authority to manage medical work without reference to the bureaucratic hierarchy, and to control the work of other health care occupations, such as nursing staff. Clearly, then, there is potential for conflict, between both the authority of hospital management, rooted in the bureaucratic hierarchy, and the attempts of other occupations to 'professionalise' and gain control over their own practice. This potential conflict, although it rarely becomes explicit (most hospitals run with an apparent consensus most of the time), has wide-ranging implications for the implementation of policy directed at the structure and role of the hospital, given that these different groups (doctors, managers, other health care workers) may have very different goals.

A negotiated order?

The question of how this apparent consensus happens is an important one. Given the potential for conflict, how do hospitals work? Work from the 1960s by Strauss and his colleagues on psychiatric hospitals in the United States (Strauss *et al* 1963) suggested that hospitals could best be described as having a 'negotiated order'. They asked the question: 'How is order maintained in the face of inevitable change?' The formal rules which exist in organisations, they argued, could never explain much about how order is achieved and maintained. Even where there are rules which govern behaviour, no one uses them all or even knows them all. Rules are more likely to be tacit expectations of behaviour than explicit formulas for decision making. Hospitals are characterised by a heterogeneous mix of professional and nonprofessional staff who may share only the most abstracted aims, such as that of improving the health of their patients. Such vague goals specify little about how this is best achieved: which treatments to use, which ward to place the patient on, how long they should stay and so on. Staff are engaged, then, in an endless cycle of negotiation over organisation. Such negotiation is patterned by the expectations different members of staff have of others, but it is not bound by formal rules.

Health care organisations in the United States: recent developments

In the United States, much has changed since Strauss and his co-workers were observing hospital organisation, and several developments have reduced the autonomy of clinicians. One is the rising interest in 'managed care' as a strategy for reducing costs (Freeborn and Pope 1994). In the United States, costs have escalated partly because there are few barriers to the use of expensive secondary facilities: there are no 'gatekeepers' in the form of a universal primary care service, such as that of the NHS (see Chapter 4). As most costs for health care are met through insurance, there are few incentives for patients or providers to reduce demands. Managed care involves introducing limits: either for patients who sign up with particular health care plans, or for providers who work for them (see Chapter 3). Doctors, for instance, in return for the ready client group that a managed care plan provides, must perhaps agree to follow cost-effective protocols for treating specified health problems. Patients who belong to the health plan must agree to see only the physicians it employs, and only to use secondary care facilities if they are referred by a primary care physician. About 14 per cent of the population in the United States are now enrolled in health maintenance organisations (HMOs) (Freeborn and Pope 1994), which provide 'managed care' in the form of providing a stated range of primary and secondary care services for payment for the plan, plus a small 'co-payment', or fee for service, each time they visit the doctor. Thus costs are reduced because patients are dissuaded from trivial attendances, and cannot self-refer to expensive hospital facilities, and physicians cannot investigate and treat without reference to the protocols of the plan. Professional autonomy over individual treatment decisions is thus eroded by managerial power.

Clinical autonomy in Britain

Although such innovations as protocols and clinical budgets are also in evidence in NHS hospitals, the explicit 'bureaucratisation' of health care organisations evident in the HMO model has not happened to the same extent. However, it has been argued that HMOs were the inspiration for the introduction of a 'managed market' to the NHS as part of the 1990 reforms (Allsop and May 1993). How far, then, has medical autonomy been eroded in favour of bureaucratic power in Britain? The role of management has certainly been strengthened by several policy initiatives over the last 25 years; first, in the early 1980s, Roy Griffiths (then a director of Sainsbury's) led an inquiry into NHS management. His report, the Griffiths' Report (DHSS 1983), advocated the introduction of general management into every layer of the NHS to replace the traditional 'consensus management' that was perceived as dominated by clinical interests. General managers, it was hoped, would provide strong leadership, effect organisational change and increase efficiency within the service.

More recently, the 1990 reforms continued the trend towards controlling clinical activity through management. The key to the 'managed market' of the new NHS is contracting, and contracting requires planning and monitoring. In crude terms, this has led to large increases in the numbers of managerial staff within the NHS: by about 260 per cent between 1989 and 1992, according to one estimate (Allsop 1995: 188). The purchasing (or commissioning) function of health authorities includes deciding which services to commission, potentially acting as constraint on clinicians' rights to determine treatment for their patients. Within the provider units, managers are responsible for providing services within budgets and ensuring that clinical activity is audited. Many hospital managers are clinicians, holding budgets for their own directorates, but these changes in the management orientation of hospitals have raised the question: to what extent has managerial power constrained professional autonomy?

Mary Ann Elston (1991) notes that during the 1960s and 1970s it was assumed that the medical profession enjoyed a monopoly of legitimacy within the health care sector, and that it had the power to block all attempts at control. However, the relative power of the profession is now more debatable, with sociologists suggesting that medicine in Britain is becoming 'deprofessionalised' or even 'proletarianised'. Elston argues that it is difficult to test these hypotheses for two reasons. First, it is difficult to operationalise concepts like 'power' and 'autonomy', especially in complex organisations such as modern hospitals. Second, many of the changes that potentially affect the position of clinicians have had too little time to take effect, and much of the academic literature is concerned with theoretical implications rather than empirical studies.

It has been noted that doctors and managers still operate from within very different value systems (Kaye and West 1986). One difference lies in their orientation towards the organisation itself. Hunter (1994) argues that although we talk about 'the profession' of medicine, it is in fact a very divided profession, with different specialties having their own royal colleges (such as the Royal College of Physicians, the Royal College of General Practitioners) and with hierarchical divisions between junior doctors and consultants. The profession, he suggests, has little corporate identity and little sense of 'belonging' to the NHS. In contrast to the individualistic orientation of doctors, managers emphasise the value of teamwork, collaboration and commitment to the wider organisation. Hunter and others (see, e.g., Mechanic 1991) have argued that clinical power is resistant to managerial encroachment for a number of reasons. A key one is the ideology of 'doctor knows best', still a powerful cultural value which legitimises the behaviour of doctors who, for instance, refuse to treat patients according to protocols. The resilience of this ideology is evident in many of the sympathetic media reports of these cases. Other sources of resistance to managerial encroachment on clinical decision making are more strategic, and include the involvement of doctors in hospital management and their control over the process of medical audit, which could otherwise be utilised as a 'tool' of management (Hunter 1994).

The potential constraints on medical power in Britain come not from the demands of bureaucratic organisations such as HMOs, but from the activities of the state, through policy designed to strengthen the management function within the NHS. However, it would be a mistake to see the encroachment of bureaucracy as inevitably leading to an erosion of professional status. As Johnson (1995) points out, although professionals portray the state as a threat to their independence, it is the state which has been integral to the constitution of medicine as a profession. Professional expertise, he argues, is central to the process of governmentality, and the profession is the state, in terms of how medicine, for instance, performs the tasks of defining health and disease and monitoring it.

At the more local level, to what extent are doctors constrained in their ability to make individual treatment decisions? There have been few empirical studies of the effects of the reforms on the division of labour on the ground, but one study by Judith Green and David Armstrong (see Box 5.2) of how different hospital staff perceive the problem of emergency admissions suggests that, at the margins at least, there has been some erosion of clinical autonomy.

Box 5.2 The organisation of emergency admissions: the erosion of clinical autonomy?

The context
In the early 1990s, emergency admissions to London hospitals had attracted attention in both professional and public media, with reports of problems in many accident and emergency departments. As a response to the problem, many hospitals had instituted a system of bed management, with a manager or team responsible for the rational allocation of patients to

beds throughout the hospital. This system potentially comes into conflict with the traditional control which consultants enjoyed over 'their' beds on hospital wards. The admission of emergency patients, in principle, is an ideal arena in which clinical autonomy would be expected to operate, as clinicians can claim that only their expertise can decide whether, and where, an admission is appropriate.

The study
Forty semistructured interviews were conducted with a range of staff (bed managers, senior accident and emergency department medical and nursing staff, general managers and other specialty consultants) with an interest in emergency admissions in nine London hospitals. In addition, three bed managers were observed through a shift. The aims were to examine perceptions of 'the problem' of emergency admissions and solutions to it.

Findings
Bed management appeared to be a successful strategy, with most staff interviewed claiming that it was a 'necessary change' and an improvement on previous mechanisms for managing the admission of emergency patients while ensuring enough beds were available for elective (nonemergency, or booked) patients. Although there were tales of resistance to bed management, from, for instance, consultants who claimed that other staff managed to 'hide' beds from managers to admit their own patients, in practice bed managers appeared to have considerable power. The bed managers themselves were careful to claim that they never 'usurped clinical autonomy', but observations and interviews suggested that in some hospitals there were situations in which managers were making decisions that did undermine those of doctors, including insisting on admission, declining admission and deciding the ward to which a patient would be admitted. How was this authority achieved?

Two rhetorics contributed to the legitimacy of bed managers. One was a rhetoric of rationality: that they had an overview of the bed stock of the whole hospital and the needs of all patients, and were therefore in a position to allocate resources in the most effective way. Related to this was a rhetoric of neutrality. Before the implementation of bed management, consultants were in conflict with other specialties over beds, and emergency patients were in conflict with those from waiting lists. The most successful bed managers had presented themselves as 'honest brokers', and other staff accepted their role as a neutral arbiter, not tied to the interests of any one specialty. A further source of legitimation was the perceived 'crisis' in beds. Although the word 'crisis' suggests a short-term problem, emergency admissions were seen to be in permanent crisis in London. The acceptance of a crisis, and a widespread belief among respondents to this survey that extra resources (such as more beds) would not help as they would merely increase demand, necessitated crisis measures. This included accepting that the bed manager could allocate patients in the most efficient way throughout the hospital, including utilising beds that were ordinarily outside the normal bed stock (such as those designated for private patients, or for particular specialties) and utilising beds irrespective of the gender, age or specialty normally taken by the ward.

Implications
There is some evidence, then, that the ideology of clinical autonomy can be undermined, at least in this particular situation. What is also of interest is the impact this had on the structure of the hospital. Bed management had created a new referent: the hospital as a whole. Whereas the ward, with its own specialty and consultants, was traditionally the focus of hospital organisation, the hospital wide remit, and practice, of bed management had legitimated the management of the hospital itself as an organisation.

Sources: Green and Armstrong 1993, 1995

This study illustrates how management is achieved on the ground: it does not just happen because of the Griffiths' Report, or because the internal market consolidates managerial practices, it has to be negotiated by individual staff in hospitals. In a wider sense, this study also perhaps suggests something about the resilience of the hospital itself as an institution. Hunter (1994: 13) argues that one source of pressure on doctors to become more managerially accountable may be the vulnerability of individual hospitals within the post-1991 internal market. As hospitals increasingly become subject to market pressure, and in competition with other providers, they will have to develop a corporate culture, he suggests, which includes professionals as well as managers. Bed management appears to be one strategy which contributes to the hospital's corporate sense.

Studying the process of management: 'bottom-up' approaches

Micro studies of organisations in hospitals, which examine the grounded practices of staff responsible for local operationalisation of policy, can offer much of interest to the policy analyst. Studies on health care arenas such as casualty reception (Hughs 1989) and the admissions office (Pope 1991) suggest that policy decision are reconstructed by 'street level bureaucrats' (Lipsky 1980), those front line staff who have responsibility for implementing bureaucratic rules. Such rules are, of course, applied with discretion, and this discretion itself forms part of informal organisation of the hospital, as the local culture by which rules are applied, ignored, elaborated or interpreted moulds the application of policy. If the study in Box 5.2 illustrated how policy was successfully implemented, and what other impacts it had, micro-level studies can also illustrate why strategic policy may not get translated into operational policy. 'Bottom-up' approaches to policy analysis focus on the local rather than the central level of policy, and draw our attention to 'discretion' in the operationalisation of policy. They also suggest some of the potential barriers to policy implementation. Qualitative sociology, particularly using methods such as participant observation, which can reveal what people do in practice, rather than what formal accounts suggest they do, has much to offer here. Box 5.3 is an example from Catherine Pope's study of admissions office clerks.

Box 5.3 Understanding NHS waiting lists with a 'bottom-up' approach.

The problem
In 1990, over one million people were waiting for treatment from NHS hospitals, and about 25 per cent of those had been waiting for more than a year for admission.

Solutions proposed
Catherine Pope points out that attempts by policy makers to remedy this problem depend on the assumptions made about how waiting lists develop and why they persist. For instance, the Department of Health's 1986 Waiting List Initiative assumed that there was a 'backlog' of untreated disease, so it funded district-level projects to clear up the backlog. The 1984 Griffiths enquiry saw waiting lists as an outcome of inefficient management. Other policy analysts conceptualise waiting lists as a 'mortlake': a pool of patients waiting for admission, particularly for certain procedures (such as hip replacements or varicose vein treatment) which command little public interest or funding.

The study

This research aimed to study how waiting lists operate on the ground – how they are produced and maintained – in order to understand why attempts to reduce them have been ineffective on the whole.

Pope addressed the problem of waiting lists from the 'bottom up', by observing the work of those staff involved in organising the waiting list and admissions to the hospital. Her approach was informed by organisation theory and the sociology of work, which suggest that informal organisations may be as important to how bureaucracies operate as formal ones. Thus, looking at the work of front line staff (in this case clerks in the admissions office of hospital in a suburban district health authority) may be crucial to understanding how health policy operates in practice.

The main findings

Clerks in the hospital admissions office were 'keepers of the queue'. They manage the waiting list on a day-to-day level, booking cases for surgeons' operating lists, notifying patients and dealing with enquiries. They had considerable discretion in their work, in terms of deciding how urgent particular cases were, organising operating lists to reflect the particular interest of individual surgeons and in deciding who would be notified to fill a cancelled admission. In summary, Pope (1991: 203) suggests that: 'Doctors and admission staff make decisions about whom to admit on the basis of professional interests, personal preferences and prejudices'. 'Personal preferences and prejudices' included the clerks' judgements about patients' deservedness, which was influenced by how willing they seemed to be to accept any date for admission and how easy they were to contact. Chance also played a part in determining how quickly patients were offered an admission date: if, for instance, the patient was lucky enough to ring just after another had cancelled.

These factors meant that the waiting list did not operate like a queue, in which clinical need would be the only criterion which affected the 'first come, first served' principle of eligibility for admission. Instead, Pope suggests that the waiting list is more usefully described as a 'store', kept by clinicians, managers and clerks, who actively manage the pool of waiting patients.

Pope's study suggests why attempts to reduce waiting lists have had limited success: they do not take into account the organisational practices which create the waiting list on the ground, and which might be quite resistant to managerial attempts to dictate policy from above.

Source: Pope 1991

What studies such as this one and the one in Box 5.2 suggest is that there is nothing inevitable about the implementation of policy. How strategic initiatives such as those directed as general management or waiting lists get put into practice is the result of local action by those responsible for implementing the new 'rules'. Those on the receiving end of policy, the patients or clients, also of course influence its effectiveness. Although strategies for 'resisting' policy shifts may be limited, there is evidence that the actions of those on the receiving end do shape the final policy, and affect its implementation. One good example is from a study which compared health visiting with therapeutic communities (Bloor and McIntosh 1990). Clients of these services, argued Bloor and McIntosh, were able to 'resist' the surveillance implicit in service delivery in a number of ways. Surveillance is essential both to the preventative services provided by health visitors (monitoring young children for abuse, assessing children's development and encouraging 'good' childcare) and to the therapeutic work of residential communities. The institutional context of health care delivery affects the type and extent of surveillance involved. Bloor and McIntosh suggest that in residential therapeutic communities, surveillance may be most extensive, and based either on direct observation or on self-reports, whereby the clients are encouraged to self-monitor their behaviour. In domiciliary based services, such as health visiting, surveillance has to be covert, or naturalistic. Given that health visitors have neither the authority nor the opportunity to examine the lives of their clients in detail, they are reliant on questioning their clients and looking around their houses when it is possible to do it unobtrusively. These techniques make possible different techniques of resistance. In therapeutic communities, where the clients are together, it is possible for 'collective ideological dissent' to occur, in which the prevailing ideology of the service is directly challenged. More common is 'individual ideological dissent', or individual clients challenging the legitimacy of the service providers. Noncompliance is also possible in both kinds of institutional context, where clients simply refuse to take part, for instance, in group work in the community, or refuse to act on the health visitor's advice. The most common form of resistance, say Bloor and McIntosh, was concealment. Clients of the health visitors, for instance, reported telling their health visitors what they wanted to hear, while continuing to behave in different ways, or simply pretending to be out when they call.

A complete account of the impact of policy needs, then, to examine not only the formal content of the policy (such as the recommendations of a White Paper), but also the implementation of that policy on the ground. Front line professionals and their clients mould the final shape of health policy even in situations where the major direction of health policy is centrally directed.

Nursing and the division of labour in hospitals

Much of the sociological debate about hospitals has centred around the relative power of managers and clinicians, and so far we have considered three groups of actors within health care organisations: managers, doctors and their patients. The main providers of patient care, however, in terms of numbers of staff, are nurses.

Nursing, gender and hierarchy

The previous section has shown how organisational theory can be used to analyse that system of health care called 'the hospital'. This section will use a different theoretical perspective, that of gender, to analyse another aspect of hospital organisation: nursing, and the doctor–nurse relationship. It is generally held that nursing has changed since the days of Sairey Gamp, the uncouth nurse in Dickens' *Martin Chuzzlewit* (first published in 1843) or Grace Poole, the drunken nurse employed to watch Mrs Rochester in Charlotte Brontë's (1847) *Jane Eyre*, or even Florence Nightingale. Nursing, since becoming a profession (the first Register was set up in 1919), has become a higher status, centrally recognised health care profession. Yet the crucial distinction remains. Nursing is not medicine and the central tension emerges: in order to be of high status the profession must lay claim to clinical and curative skills, but in order to remain as 'nursing' the practice must be centred on caring for, not curing patients.

Nursing's professional bodies are caught in a double bind: how to improve the status (and therefore rewards) of nursing without losing its patient-centred role? This has in part been addressed by the conscious formation of a body of theoretical knowledge, the nursing process (Macfarlane 1977), particular to nursing and distinct from medicine, which will form the basis of its claim to separate disciplinary status (as has health promotion, see Chapter 2). This has to some extent been the rationale behind the more recent developments in nurse education; for example, the creation of Project 2000 (UKCC 1986) and the possibility of a degree in nursing, which superseded the old apprentice style ward-based training of 'pupil' nurses. This change marks the shift in site from hospital to college and from 'training' to 'education'. Are these changes simply part of an ongoing battle between doctors and nurses for recognition and status? Or are they a response to the new management structure where outside managers have replaced nurses in the hospital's administrative structure, thus reducing their power and influence in the hospital organisation? The explanation may, however, go beyond either of these policy-based issues and be seen as a gender issue, which will be explored further here. The history of nursing, that is, the formation of policies which create the domain of nursing, serves as an illustration of how gender categories are produced.

Historically, the shift from home to hospital was important for the development of the clinical gaze and this was discussed earlier in this chapter and in relation to public health in Chapter 2. As has been well documented elsewhere, scientific medicine's gaze shifted from the whole person, to the body, to lesions, then cells and pathology (Foucault, quoted in Burchell *et al.* 1987; Armstrong 1983). The concept of epidemiology (and the use of invader metaphors) appeared with the increase of poor urban populations and medical institutions became concerned with the mapping of contagion. This was, for example, expressed in the Contagious Diseases Acts of the 1860s which sought to regulate women's sexuality. (The laws were to apply to naval towns where the prostitutes were held to be responsible for seducing men and contributing to the increase in sexually transmitted disease; this is discussed in relation to contemporary law on HIV/AIDS by Mort 1987, see discussion in Chapter 2.)

Medicine, nursing and professonalisation

As discussed earlier in this chapter, this shift to a 'scientific basis' for medicine was part of the move to professionalisation, marked by the setting up of the GMC and the regulation of entry to the profession, which formally excluded women and, in the USA, 'blacks'. These changes sought to regulate the numbers of practitioners (thus ensuring a living for the chosen few). This exclusionary practice was particularly marked in the USA where wealthy philanthropists like Rockefeller and Carnegie, in their (successful) attempts to stay at the leading edge of the new, and potentially profitable, developments in 'scientific medicine', were funding medical schools for white males only. We have, perhaps unwittingly, become familiar with the effects of this through the stereotype figures of the Wild West: with the travelling 'quacks', practitioners unable to register and trying to earn a living by selling their 'water of life' at the roadside and the 'Doc Holliday' figure from TV westerns, whose drinking and other social practices would fall foul of any code of professional conduct.

In Britain, the Victorian constructions of upper-class femininity ensured that women were considered unsuitable candidates for higher education in general and the GMC merely enshrined in its regulations what had been, with a few notable exceptions, usual practice anyway.

This particular legislation created the formal gendered division of labour apparent in contemporary health care. Women have, of course, always been central to the provision of health care (Stacey 1988; Pelling 1983) and the divide between caring and curing has not always been so clearly marked. The village wise women of the Middle Ages with a knowledge of herbs and midwifery were those who could provide practical interventions into ordinary people's lives. The physicians were able only to pray for the sick and to provide bedside comfort and spiritual support. Perhaps the first policy of major significance regulating the role of women in health care occurred during the thirteenth century. The Church's domination and regulation of the practice of medicine legally precluded women from the university training necessary to qualify for the profession. Women healers were subsequently sought out and condemned as heretics, or witches.

These 'witch hunts' acted to prevent women providing healing and midwifery services for ordinary women and attempted to restrict healing to physicians and clergymen. It is no coincidence that the women accused of witchcraft were often unmarried and economically independent, this, as we shall see, remains a problem in contemporary nursing:

> . . . lay healers of this period were empiricists; they believed in
> trial and error, cause and effect. This was the very opposite of the
> Church's position, which opposed the value of the material world,
> distrusting any emphasis on knowledge obtained via the senses.
> The Church attacked the 'magic' of the lay healer through the
> institutions of the witch hunt. Clearly other issues were involved.
> Approximately 85 per cent of 'witches' denounced and punished
> by the Church were women and in addition to being charged
> with the use of healing and midwifery skills, female witches were

accused of committing sexual crimes against men and of possessing
a 'female sexuality'. As Ehrenreich and English [1973] point out,
the persecution of witches represented not only the anti-empiricist
but also the anti-sexual obsessions of the Church at this time.

(Savage 1987: 63–4)

A suitable job for a woman?

Nursing, as opposed to healing, was a less contentious sphere as
it was seen as an extension of women's domestic role. As a consequence no special skills were deemed necessary for it and it
became the domain of working-class women who were not caring
for a family of their own. The reputation of these women was as
drunken and untrustworthy (again a stereotype often applied to
women who have an identity outside of that of wife and mother
in a heterosexual nuclear family), and nursing was not a job for
respectable women.

However, nursing as a paid occupation for middle-class women
arose during the nineteenth century largely as a result of the
professionalisation of medicine and its barring of women but also
partly due to a demographic change which resulted in 'an excess
of spinsters'. 'Respectable' women who could not be married were
able instead to find financial security in an occupational sphere
deemed acceptable, for example, as a governess or as a nurse.

These were the factors behind Florence Nightingale's cam-
paigning for the recognition of 'the nurse' as a suitable job for
a (middle-class) woman. The story has it that she deliberately
did not suggest that nurses were equivalent to doctors as a way of
ensuring support for her plans from the professional medical men.
Similarly, to counter criticisms that it was 'unnatural', Nightingale
proposed that to be a good nurse was to be a good woman;
indeed, this sentiment was echoed in a DHSS recruitment advert
in the early 1980s, where the caption under a picture of a small
girl dressed in a 'nurse's uniform' read 'The best nurses have
the essential qualifications before they go to school' (Smith 1992).
Thus by the end of the nineteenth century medicine and nursing
had divided into two separate professions, each profoundly
gendered.

As described in the first part of this chapter, the end of the
nineteenth century also saw the development of the hospital as an
organisation. This put nurses (and therefore women) into the public sphere. A strategy for managing this anomaly was the familial

analogy which operated, with the doctor as 'husband and father', the nurse as 'wife and mother' and the patient as child:

> The ideal nurse was a transformation of the ideal lady. Relieved of her reproductive responsibilities, she was transposed from domestic life to hospital life, taking with her her wifely obedience to the doctor (who was in turn the perfect gentleman) and motherly concern for the patient. Nursing came 'naturally to women, second only to motherhood'.
>
> (Savage 1987: 66)

These 'relationships' remain central to the way the hierarchy of health professions are constructed.

Take, for example, the case of midwifery during the nineteenth century. Then, childbirth took place largely in the home and was attended by midwives, a female occupation, which at that stage was unregistered. But 'difficult' or abnormal labours were moved into hospitals where men could make 'medical interventions'. It was at this point that 'obstetrics' as a medical specialty was created. Clearly these doctors could not also be called midwives and the term 'obstetrics' (meaning 'to stand in front of') was used to differentiate this practice. The midwives consolidated their position as a nursing profession with the 1902 Midwives Act which obliged all practicing midwives to be registered. Midwives were also legally obliged to have an obstetrician attend any 'abnormal' births. This remains the case, although since the 1970s childbirth outside of hospital has become the exception (and requires the birth to be both normal and in the presence of a doctor).

Doctors and nurses, men and women

This sort of differentiation is also typical of the relationship between nurses and doctors within the hospital organisation. Nurses' technical activities are regulated by what doctors allow them to do:

> For example, medical advancement and specialisation have so complicated individual practice that physicians have been forced to relinquish tasks to subordinate or technical personnel.
>
> (Pape 1978: 65)

Indeed, by 1948 17 former doctors' tasks had become the responsibility of nurses (Pape 1978: 66). This included the use of the thermometer, which had been considered too technical for nurses. At this point thermometers were considered 'low tech' and doctors had moved on to higher status, more technical things:

Initially, such tasks would be carried out by the doctor or his students. After the innovatory stage, however, such a use of doctors became increasingly unattractive since there was a lack of novelty and an apparent waste of painfully acquired skills on what were now routine tasks.

(Dingwall and McIntosh 1978: 37)

Similarly, it was common for men practising as GPs to marry nurses, often training at the same hospital, who could be relied upon to run the surgery, which until the 1960s was usually a couple of rooms in their own home. This is also true of dentistry, where GDPs' wives were often hygienists or dental nurses and they both practised out of the family home. It was commonly accepted that middle-class girls would train as nurses in the expectation that they would meet and marry a doctor (and they frequently did). This sexualising of the power dynamic is a frequent theme in romantic fiction, itself a product of the liberal age. In these stories the power of the nurse/ woman comes from being needed (by men) (see, for example the Mills and Boon romances). It is worth considering these stereotypes of nurses and doctors.

There are a number of stereotypes of male and female nurses. There is the madonna/whore dyad for single women: respectively illustrated by the TV series 'Angels' (and indeed in almost any nursing drama over the last 40 years) and Barbara Windsor in the 'Carry On' movies; and the 'Matron', a (hetero)sexually repressed, usually ugly, often upper middle-class, older woman (for example Hattie Jacques in the 'Carry On' movies). This is sometimes countered by the 'maternal type' of older woman who is approachable but neither sexy (as unavailable) or powerful.

The madonna/whore ambiguity which characterises the stereotypes of 'the nurse' are akin to the positionings available within contemporary culture for all single heterosexual women. We might see this as a strategy for keeping women who are in positions of economic and social independence in subordinate gender positions. This is demonstrated by the reported behaviours of many male patients towards female nurses. These encounters are often flirtatious, an exercising of heterosexual masculinity acting to restore the 'rightful' power dynamic between the incapacitated man and the autonomous woman. Similarly, many nurses can relate to stories of male patients leaving their pyjamas undone when walking about the ward.

Jocelyn Lawler (1991), in her study of how nurses manage 'the body' in their work, discusses the embarrassment of female nurses having to wash male bodies being more than that of male nurses having to wash female bodies: 'The power invested in the male body is a theme which occurs throughout this study' (p. 118). Nurses have to 'work' at making a bed bath a 'nursing' task not a sexualised one, through various strategies they learn such as emotional detachment and creating a clinical atmosphere. They report problems with men who break the accepted rules and behave as if it were a sexual encounter (Lawler 1991: 196–8). Female nurses in the study reported that sexual behaviour from men was a common occurrence (pp. 203–6), which reflected the way in which nurses are constructed by society. Lawler suggests that the nursing ideology of caring, in which the professional nurse should be able to care for any patient, no matter how difficult, prevents this from being constructed as sexual harassment (p. 208).

The construction of nurses as 'sexy' also has the effect of ruling out the possibility of the lesbian nurse (depicted as hatchet faced, cruel and humourless – see for example 'Big Nurse' in the film of Ken Kesey's novel, *One Flew over the Cuckoo's Nest*, directed by Miles Foreman 1975) whilst at the same time enabling any woman refusing to play the 'flirtation' game to be 'kept in line' through 'jokes', insults or whispered speculations.

The male patient also demands a particular interaction with any male nurse. As nursing is equated with caring, and caring with femininity, any man in this role is by definition acting outside the discourse of masculinity, and therefore perceived as gay. Thus heterosexual men being cared for (rather than cured) by men will need to assert their masculine identity by actively displaying their heterosexuality, for example, discussing sport, which (female) nurses are attractive, and so on. Equally, men in nursing will be constructed in their heterosexual masculinity by becoming the romantic object of the (heterosexual) women they work amongst, thus making their relationships with male patients 'safe'.

The exception to this is in psychiatric nursing, where nurses are deemed to need physical strength to manage potentially difficult patients, in which cases nurses are presumed to be male.

Indeed in mainstream nursing very few men remain at the practitioner level. Men in nursing are far more likely than their female equivalents to achieve management posts. According to Davies and Rosser (1986) women in nursing took significantly longer than men to be promoted to a senior nursing post, even when they had not taken a career break. Salvage, writing in 1985, documents:

... there is only about one male to every 19 female nursing
auxiliaries and assistants (1980 figures, England only) ... In senior
jobs ... nearly half the top management and education posts [are]
occupied by men.

(Salvage 1985: 35)

Thus despite the entry of increased numbers of men to the profession in recent years (the GNC only documented this between
1955 and 1971, during which time the percentage of men rose from
approximately 5 per cent to 10 percent of the nursing workforce)
the male nurse remains an anomaly.

The nurse/doctor binary pair are perceived as forming a complementary whole, mirroring the ideal type heterosexual couple:

Medicine and nursing came to be seen as complementary activities
in the sense that if nursing was feminine, medicine was masculine:
the nurse was the ideal woman, the doctor the ideal man. His
intelligent, active, pragmatic, qualities were appropriate for the
aggressive treatment of disease but not compatible with caring.

(Savage 1987: 66)

Nurses are, therefore, caring, nurturing, intuitive, domestic, pretty
and feminine, whilst doctors are tough, decisive, rational, clever
and masculine. Thus women are nurses and doctors are men.

Prospects for the future

It is a matter of speculation as to how these patterns will alter with
the increase of numbers of women in the professions of medicine
and dentistry. Since the beginning of the 1990s approximately equal
numbers of young men and women have been entering medical
and dental schools. It is possible that this will lead to a gradual
change in the hierarchy, as by default more women will be available to be selected for senior hospital posts, and a subtle change
in the culture where it will be expected that doctors and dentists
are as likely to be women as men; it will no longer be necessary to
talk of the 'lady doctor'. Another scenario is also possible: that
medicine and dentistry will follow the pattern of teaching as a
profession. Where teaching was once a high status profession
occupied by men, teachers now, particularly in primary schools,
are predominantly women and the status of teaching has declined.
Where men remain in teaching it is in the relatively higher status
secondary schools and disproportionately in senior management
positions. The unequal distribution of women amongst medical

and dental specialties is already well-documented (Webster 1993; Seward and McEwan 1987); it could be that as the proportion of women becoming doctors and dentists increases, the status of the profession will decrease, leaving the men to fill the prestigious senior hospital positions and with the majority of women working in general practice.

'Race' and the nursing hierarchy

Just as there is a clear gender hierarchy in health care professions, so there are clear divisions along lines of ethnicity. The NHS is the largest employer of black and minority ethnic people in the UK, yet the evidence is that they are disproportionately represented in the lower grades of every strata. The unequal access of minority ethnic doctors to higher status medical specialties is well-documented (Smith 1980), although there is no comparable literature on dentistry. However, this divide also exists within nursing, with women from black and minority ethnic backgrounds being more likely to be found in the auxiliary grades. This too fits with the stereotype of black women as suited to 'servant' or 'domestic' roles and perhaps even more offensively as 'less sensitive', and in racist ideology, less developed (in an evolutionary sense) and so less suited to the caring role of nursing.

During the 1960s, as part of the postwar reconstruction and expansion of the health service, there was a mass recruitment of Caribbean and Irish nurses to the NHS. Recruitment offices were set up in the Caribbean and personal letters were sent to many potential recruits, encouraging them to come and help build a better Britain. The Health Minister between 1961–3 was Enoch Powell, later made infamous by his antipathy towards nonwhite immigration (and in particular his inflammatory 'rivers of blood' speech in 1968). The irony of personally having received a letter of invitation to this country from Enoch Powell has not been lost on these people.

Many African-Caribbean nurses were encouraged to sign up for SEN (State Enrolled Nurse) rather than SRN (State Registered Nurse) training without it being made explicit that this was a 'second rate' qualification with limited career progression and that the possibility of transferring to SRN was remote (Bryan et al. 1985). Thus there is a gender and a race hierarchy within and between every strata of health care and this both produces, and is produced by, the emergence of particular health care polices.

De-institutionalisation: community care

Local hospitals are usually the object of considerable community support, in evidence whenever there are threats to close one. However, hospitals also engender rather ambivalent feelings in those who have to stay in them, and it is not very long ago that the workhouse origins of many hospital buildings were part of local folk tradition. In the introduction to her book on the Anatomy Act, Ruth Richardson recalls:

> As a child in the mid-50s in London's Notting Hill, I can clearly remember the local belief that the chimney of a nearby hospital (an old work house infirmary) belched the smoke of human fuel. In my school playground small children nodded knowingly, and told each other that those who went in there never came out.
>
> (Richardson 1989: xvi)

Although the dread associated with the workhouse may have subsided, much of the research which has focused on the patient's experience of hospitals has highlighted the negative effects of institutionalisation. This has been particularly apparent in the area of long-term psychiatric care.

The rise and decline of asylums

Andrew Scull (1983) has detailed how psychiatric care became 'medicalised' as the state became increasingly involved in directly controlling institutions for deviant members of the community. The development of institutions segregating different kinds of deviants (criminals, the insane, those incapable of work) from their communities was a relatively recent development in Europe and the United States, he argues, where the control of deviants was generally a community affair until the late eighteenth century. Only since then have asylums, which made possible the development of the 'helping' professions, been a feature of social control.

For Scull, the development of asylums as a solution to the problem of what to do with the insane is intricately tied to the development of capitalist relations of production and a commercialisation of social life, which disrupted traditional ties of obligation between the rich and poor. The discipline and routine of the asylum, like other institutions of social control (the prison, the workhouse) was a route for instilling factory work habits into those outside the labour force. During the nineteenth century, asylums expanded and became enormous institutions, with a largely lower-class clientele. The marginal status of inmates meant that psychiatry did not enjoy much prestige during the nineteenth century, when the asylum was primarily an institution of social control rather than curing or caring. By the middle of the twentieth century, the asylum had come under considerable scrutiny as a health care institution. One classic study of the impact of hospitals on those who stay in them was Erving Goffman's (1961) study of long-stay psychiatric hospitals in the USA, *Asylums*. Goffman used participant observation to gather data on how the institution impacted on patient's behaviour and their sense of 'self'. For Goffman these hospitals were an example of a 'total institution', which controlled all aspects of the life of an inmate. Separated from the outside world, psychiatric inpatients are completely subordinated to the routines of the hospital, which dictate when they eat, who they socialise with, and how they dress. All information about the individual becomes the property of the institution, which can pass it between staff. The patient has to develop an institutional 'self' who complies with the rules of the hospital and which eventually completely encroaches on identity.

Goffman's work is part of the 'cultural backdrop' which influenced public opinion and policy makers concerned about the effect of long-term care on those living in institutions. However, many other factors have been suggested for the declining numbers of psychiatric patients in large institutions (a process Scull has labelled 'decarceration') from the middle of the twentieth century. One possible explanation is the development of new forms of treatment, such as psychotropic drugs, which enable people to be treated outside an institution. Scull (1977) and many others are critical of this explanation, given that numbers began falling before the widespread use of such drugs. Again, Scull (1977) focuses more on economic explanations: that large-scale asylums became too expensive for the state to run. Lindsay Prior (1991) examines the shift in policy as a result of changes in the discourses of psychiatry, which focus on therapy and the connection of the individual with society, which are incompatible with institutional life. Much of the research we have highlighted in this chapter has looked at how health care organisations impact on medical knowledge and the delivery of care: Prior's argument is interesting because he examines the ways in which knowledge can impact on organisation. In the late twentieth century, he argues, responsibility for mental illness is widely dispersed, with input from social services, doctors, nurses and a variety of other therapists. Nursing approaches, for example, are based on holistic models of care, in which the relationships a patient has and the ways in which they manage 'activities of daily living' are viewed as interdependent. The rise of such nursing models, at the expense of a focus on disease and diagnostic labels, has brought with it an inevitable focus beyond the hospital ward and into the community.

Before looking at the content of 'decarceration' policy in Britain, it is worth pointing out two caveats to the argument that long-term institutions are damaging for patients. One is that this is not inevitable. Pauline Prior (1995), in a case study of an Irish man from a long-term hospital, shows how the combination of a strong personal identity that predated hospital admission and an institution which is broadly accepted by the local community meant that he maintained a 'self' that was not solely the result of institutional socialisation. A second caveat is that the very features which Goffman attributes to the organisation of the hospital can be apparent in other settings. Hilary Gavilan (1992) for instance, discusses her experience of caring for elderly housebound people in the light of her reading of Goffman, and concludes that many of the negative aspects of institution occur in the home, including loss of privacy, loss of control over daily routine and a loss of autonomy. We will return to the disadvantages of 'community care' below.

By the 1980s in Britain, there were strong claims made from various actors in the policy community that 'something had to be done' to provide better care in the community for people with long-term needs. The Audit Commission published its critical review of care for the mentally ill, *Making a Reality out of Community Care*, in 1986, and the DHSS published a report by Roy Griffiths on the problems in the service in 1988 (DHSS 1988). One concern was that there were a number of 'perverse incentives' which made it financially advantageous for local authorities to provide long-term institutional care rather than support in the community.

Many of the recommendations of these reports were put into practice in the 1989 White Paper *Caring for People* (DOH 1989), which became part of the 1990 NHS and Community Care Act. Like the reforms for the health sector, those for social services outlined in *Caring for People* advocated a split between purchasing and providing functions of local authorities, who would become responsible for funds to purchase care for the elderly and those with special needs currently in residential care. Individual care managers would purchase packages of care on behalf of their clients, from a mixture of public, private and voluntary organisations. It was envisaged that they would find services which enabled people to live in their own homes ('the community') when possible. The budget for meeting this need is now capped, whereas before costs for residential homes came from social security funds. This creates potential problems for local authorities unable to meet all needs in their areas. As local authorities are responsible for social, but not medical, needs there are also potential problems with implementing co-ordinated care for groups who need it most: a plethora of different agencies may be involved with the care of one elderly person.

The concept of community

Perhaps one of the biggest problems with the implementation of community care as a policy is the rather nebulous concept of 'community'. 'Community' embodies the notion of shared goals and values, of everyone working together. It has been used in policy terms to evoke the opposite of the term 'institution', which has come to symbolise remote, impersonal, detachment. 'Care', too, has complex meanings and usage. Alone it symbolises humanitarian values: to care for someone is seen as a way of expressing love and tenderness; but to be 'in care' is not redolent with such warm overtones: instead 'in care' is more equivalent to 'institution' in that it conjures up state-organised services which do not, almost by definition, care for or about people. These issues are well summarised by this passage from Means and Smith:

> But where does the positive power of the term 'community care'
> come from? Baron and Haldane argue that it flows from the fact
> that 'community is what Raymond Williams (1976) calls a keyword
> in the development of culture and society. From the ninth century
> BC through to the present time, Williams is able to trace the use
> of the term 'community' to lament the recent passing of a series
> of mythical Golden Ages. Each generation perceives the past
> as organic and whole compared to the present. As Baron and
> Haldane point out, the term 'community' thus enables 'the
> continuous construction of an idyllic past of plenty and social
> harmony which acts as an immanent critique of contemporary
> social relations' (p. 4). Thus the call by politicians and policy
> makers to replace present systems of provision with community
> care feeds into this myth by implying that it is possible to recreate
> what many believe were the harmonious, caring and integrated
> communities of the past.
>
> (Means and Smith 1994: 5)

Thus, care for those people labelled 'dependent' has become polarised into what Dalley describes as: 'Competing ideologies upon which alternative social policies for the provision of care for dependent people are based, namely familism and collectivism' (1996: 1). Which ideology, and which sort of social policy, is constructed is a consequence of the political values of the time. Currently we see an emphasis on holistic models of health care where individuals and their problems are deemed best treated as part of their whole social context, not isolated in 'specialist' facilities (that is, a familial rather than a collectivist model). Of course all these options are redolent with implicit values about what is (currently) socially desirable and what is 'normal' in terms of the social system which will support them. As Dalley goes on to say:

> Underlying much of the discussion about community care and the policies that promote it have been some fundamental assumptions about the nature and structure of family life, about the role of the family, the role of the state, and about the relative values of privacy, independence and interdependence.
>
> (Dalley 1996: 7)

These ideas of relative dependence/independence are discussed later in this chapter in relation to disability issues.

Dalley (1996: 8–11) identifies three main criticisms of the current community care policies. First, the manner in which policies are being implemented: that is, that they are largely a matter of political will and resources and have, in the past at least, been seen as a relatively cheap option in comparison to the costs of institutional care. Indeed, several political reasons have been offered as reasons for the delay in implementing the 1990 Act:

> The NHS and Community Care Act was passed by Parliament in summer 1990, only for the government to announce major delays in the implementation timetable . . . There were several possible explanations for these delays. Were they a sensible reaction to the failure of local authorities to prepare adequately for the changes? . . . were the delays an attempt to control local government expenditure because of sensitivities about the then poll-tax based system of local government finance? Or did the Conservatives wish to abandon local authorities as the lead agents in community care, if and when they won the next election?
>
> (Means and Smith 1994: 59)

The second criticism Dalley identifies is regarding the substance of the policies themselves; that is that not all 'dependencies' are equally amenable to community care and community care is often practitioner/policy maker-defined, not client-led.

The third criticism relates to the principles on which policies are based, that is that privacy and independence are desired and achievable only within a 'family', the suggestion being that caring is essentially a private business. This latter criticism clearly has implications for those who are deemed to have responsibility for the care of 'dependent people', the 'carers', of whom most are women (Graham 1986).

There has been a great deal of discussion about the effect of these policies on women, who bear the majority of the responsibility for domestic labour, and the assumptions embedded in the policy about women's role in social, political and economic life. It has also assumed, not only the desirability, but also the prevalence, of heterosexual nuclear families.

Disability and dependency

What have only recently come to be addressed are the embedded assumptions about the nature of 'disability' and the relationship between disability and dependence. Oliver (1993) and others have argued cogently in recent years that 'dependency' is a condition which applies to all human beings, but that dependency upon mobility or communication aids, for example, within certain parameters (e.g. lifts, telephones) is defined as 'normal', whilst dependency on aids outside this range (wheelchairs, hearing aids, etc.) defines the user as having a disability.

Similarly, there is a distinction between 'caring about' and 'caring for'. By extension, then, we all benefit from 'care', particularly in the sense of 'caring about', but we do not necessarily need 'caring for' in a paternalistic sense. This point is made forcibly by Morris (1993) who argues that disabled people do not seek 'care'; rather they require personal assistance or support and definitely not on a collective basis, as the memories of institutions into which disabled people were put are too painfully recent (Dalley 1996: 127). Indeed, activists in the disability movement have challenged the whole concept of 'carers' and the needs of carers as just one more way of creating disabled people's dependency; instead they argue for financial and economic autonomy and the right to choose what kind of support is purchased with their state benefits and allowances:

> Disabled people see an ideological collusion between policy makers
> and carers, which again focuses on the notion of disabled people
> as dependent, as burdens, as encroaching on the freedom and
> autonomy of those upon whom they are dependent.
>
> (Dalley 1996: 126)

It is important, however, to recognise the heterogeneity of disability and dependency and the very real differences that this can make to the kind of service provision required; whilst 'independent living' may indeed be entirely appropriate for young, relatively fit individuals, the kind of support needed for those who are 'frail' might be quite different. It is also worth considering the possibility of 'collective care'; whilst this is currently associated with state-run institutions of the worst kind, it is possible that a collectivity, that is a group of people with shared aims and values who all benefit equally from the giving and receiving of care, could be construed as a more egalitarian manner of service provision. This would be more akin to self-help groups. Whilst specialist provision, particularly for those with learning difficulties or mental illness, has had the reputation of being a 'dumping ground' or a 'ghetto', it is possible to conceive of it as being targeted provision where people with similar experiences of the world are able to give reciprocal support and friendship to one another in an environment in which they are valued. This is similar to the arguments within other social minorities for the right and need to organise separately from the mainstream 'oppressors'.

Currently services are inequitable, relying on a piecemeal and fragmented mix of voluntary and statutory provision operating in what Dalley calls 'a mutual policy and planning vacuum' (p. 145) and where access may depend on ability to pay. Also there is 'an almost total absence of non-sexist options' (Dalley 1996: 145) and this is likely to remain the case whilst social policy does not ascribe to an explicitly feminist agenda with its concomitant non-sexist philosophies and structures.

This chapter has taken a wide-ranging view on the organisation of health care both within and without the institution of the hospital. Tracing these developments has allowed us to see the emergence of health policies as part of more general transformations in forms of political power. The current trend towards 'care in the community' can therefore be seen as part of the shift towards the more diffuse forms of monitoring and surveillance identified in Chapter 2.

Exercises

Exercise 1
Compare adverts in the Yellow Pages for old peoples' homes and note the kinds of services they offer. What seem to be the priorities? Are any health or personal social services provided?

Can you infer from this anything about how 'care in the community' actually works?

Exercise 2
Carry out some observation of health care workers in a local heath centre/hospital. Are there any noticeable differences in the race and gender roles?

Exercise 3
Suggest some advantages and disadvantages of an increase in community-based health care?

What might be some of the possible implications of the increase in female medical and dental graduates for the hierarchy of health care professionals?

How might the increasing role of primary health care impact on the organisation of the hospital?

Further reading

On the organisation of the NHS
Strong, P. and Robinson, J. (1990) *The NHS: Under New Management,* Milton Keynes: Open University Press.

An empirical study, based on interviews, of what the introduction of general management meant for managers and others in the NHS.

On professions
Stacey, M. (1988) *The Sociology of Health and Healing,* London: Routledge.

A detailed and readable sociological account of the rise of biomedicine and the division of labour in modern medical care, which takes a social constructivist and feminist approach. Stacey traces the historical development of healing systems and the medical profession in Britain, from the seventeenth century to the establishment of the NHS and looks at the position of patients, unpaid carers, alternative practitioners and nurses as well as doctors in the division of labour.

Gabe, J., Kelleher, D. and Williams, G. (eds) (1994) *Challenging Medicine*, London: Routledge.

Chapters examine various threats to the professional autonomy of medicine, including those from management, law, nursing, alternative medicine, lay knowledge and self-help groups.

On community care

Means, R. and Smith, R. (1994) *Community Care: Policy and Practice*, London: Macmillan.

A very comprehensive account of the development and implementation of 'community care'.

Chapter 6

Researching health policy

Summary: This chapter looks at the issues raised, both theoretical and methodological, by doing health policy research. In the first part of this chapter we outline the funding and organisation of social science research in health policy, and the ethical and practical implications for researchers. We then address some of the main theoretical/political perspectives which have informed health policy and our understanding of it during the twentieth century. The final sections consider some of the methodological approaches used by sociologists interested in health policy analysis at the levels of outcome and process in two main areas: the elicitation of user's views and researching health services.

Introduction

Traditionally, when writing up a study, theoretical and methodological aspects are dealt with early on, as soon as the introduction has laid out the rationale for the project. In this book we have decided that questions of methodological approach and their theoretical underpinnings are best understood after the reader has had the opportunity to become familiar with some of the substantive issues. Hopefully, where particular theoretical and methodological approaches have been an integral part of the issue under discussion or the relevant case study, this will have been drawn to the readers' attention and cross-referenced to this chapter.

Much policy making rests on implicit assumptions, for example, that human need is universal and that it should be met, or that women are more naturally suited to caring, and each of these derive from particular sets of beliefs about the world and will influence the type of action (i.e. policies) which are aspired to, if not achieved. Thus, it is stating the obvious to say that policies are the result of politics, that is, systematic ideas about how society does (or should) function.

Comparing health care systems

This book has been primarily about health policy in Britain, and has used issues raised about providing the National Health Service to illustrate how sociology can help understand policy. Another level of analysis to consider is that of structure, or the macro questions that are asked about health care policy. Here, international comparisons are of great benefit, as they allow us to question taken-for-granted assumptions about the ways in which health care systems are organised. International comparisons can also be useful in understanding some of the more macro-level questions about financing health care and the role of the state. In his account of President Clinton's attempted reforms of the United States health care system, for instance, Donald Light (1994) makes some useful observations which have a bearing on evaluating the likely impact of Britain's 1990 reforms. First, he says, 'managed care' (see Chapter 5) and market forces have not driven down health care costs in the United States, as had been hoped by politicians. President Reagan's approach, like that of Margaret Thatcher, had been one of minimal state intervention and faith in the ability of competition to reduce expenditure. However, between 1980 and 1990, US expenditure on health care had risen from 9.2 per cent of GDP to 12.1 per cent. Managed care plans have resulted in individuals having to pay increasing proportions of their health care costs as direct charges, in addition to their insurance premiums. Additionally, claims Light, an ever-increasing proportion of US citizens are underinsured or not insured at all. Managed care plans, a significant influence on the 'internal market' model of the 1990 NHS reforms, are likely to maintain high costs in the long term, as they establish themselves as the most powerful health care providers in a locality and drive out the competition.

International comparisons have also been used to put the debate about resourcing the NHS into perspective. Many commentators have claimed that the NHS has been chronically underfunded, since its inception (see the Appendix). The 1990 NHS reforms attempted to solve the problems of the NHS through organisational change, without identifying extra resources to meet rising demands on its services. Johnson (1990: 89–91) argues that although the Conservative government claimed to have spent more on the NHS in real terms, this spending did not compensate for growing costs for labour, new medical technology and the fact that health care costs rise faster than the retail price index, which is usually used as the measure of inflation to compare spending over time. He cites spending compared with other countries as evidence that the NHS is comparatively underfunded: health care in Britain accounts for 6 per cent of GDP, compared with more than 8 per cent in Canada, France, Germany and Sweden.

As we have seen already, international comparisons are useful in analysing the style of national health policies, as well as their likely implications. In Chapter 2, the case study in Box 2.2 suggested that the more 'individualistic' approach of health promotion in Britain compared with Sweden results from cultural differences in the two countries' orientations towards collective responsibility and the role of the state. Another example comes from a study of HIV testing policy. Renée Danziger (1996) discusses the policy of compulsory testing for HIV in Hungary as the result of the specific social, economic and cultural conditions in the country at the time when public health doctors had to respond to early indications of an AIDS epidemic. The policy of compulsory testing persists, despite a widespread international public health consensus against such testing on the grounds that it 'drives the disease underground' and provides no benefits for those tested. Danziger argues that a consideration of the particular conditions of Hungary justify its use there, given that state-run health services mean that most infected individuals are identified through testing and provided with good quality health care once identified. Thus the 'liberal consensus' that compulsory testing is unworkable and unethical is not a statement of universal principle, but an outcome of particular circumstances.

Before moving on to looking at how such different theoretical and political perspectives influence sociological approaches, it is worth outlining the context of social research in health policy. An initial consideration is the organisation of health policy research: how it is commissioned and carried out.

The social organisation of health policy research

Research for health policy: the historical context

There are perhaps two historical contexts for understanding the role of modern health policy research. One is the growth of the state's machinery for monitoring its population, already discussed in Chapters 2 and 4. By the end of the nineteenth century, the Registrar General's office in England and Wales was collating a large number of statistics about the health of the population. The growing activities of the state required more and more facts to inform it, and the history of the state's direct involvement with research is an empirical tradition, one which has been concerned primarily with fact gathering to inform policy makers. This work continues today, in the work of the Office for National Statistics (formerly the Office for Population Censuses and Surveys), which carries out the national census every 10 years as well as other large surveys and ad hoc research.

The other tradition conventionally given as an antecedent to organised research in Britain is that of 'social reform': the tradition of marshalling facts to improve society, first evident in philanthropic studies by Victorian reformers such as the Webbs, founders of the Fabian Society; Charles Booth, the statistician and social reformer; and Ernest Chadwick, who published his *Report on the Sanitary Conditions of the Labouring Population* in 1842. This report described the appalling conditions endured by the urban poor and also outlined the inability of government to tackle these problems. Victorian social enquiry was specifically orientated towards social problems and their amelioration. This 'reforming' tradition is still a strong one in sociological research, and as we noted in Chapter 1, it is often a primary motive for doing research for policy analysis.

However, this kind of research, which is explicitly carried out to have a direct influence on policy, has had rather low status compared with more theoretical research in the social sciences. Policy-relevant research is often carried out by those with no social science training, such as researchers in government departments who have learned on the job, while researchers based in the higher education sector ('professional sociologists') have traditionally focused on 'pure' or theoretical research.

There are, however, some very good reasons why sociologists are becoming more involved with policy-orientated research in areas such as health. One practical reason is the restrictions on funding for pure research, which have encouraged researchers to turn their attentions to what will get funded: the projects with some clear relevance to the policy questions of the day. Social research skills are in much demand in the health sector, with its growing emphasis on both consumer responsiveness (which entails finding out what people want from their health services) and evaluation. Whatever your motivations for doing research, there is usually a need to find both funding and some, however minimal, institutional support. Also, perhaps just as importantly, given that results do not officially exist until they are published, it will be much easier to get papers published if there are some policy implications from your work.

As well as the pragmatic reasons for considering policy implications, there have also been calls from within the discipline for a more involved social science. One well-cited advocate was the sociologist C. Wright Mills (1959), who argued that sociologists have a responsibility not only to describe and analyse the world in their research, but also to suggest how to change that world. Sociology should be, he said, neither 'grand theory', which was irrelevant to the everyday problems that afflict people and societies, but nor should it be 'abstracted empiricism', the gathering of data merely for its own sake. In short, he suggested that sociological research should address real problems in ways which might offer solutions to those problems: what we might call policy-orientated research.

Janet Finch (1986) claims that the most compelling reason for engaging in policy-orientated research is that it is impossible to avoid it. Social scientists are, she notes, inevitably part of the social world which they study, and the knowledge that they produce will, or at least can be, used, whether they intend it to be or not. It is, she argues, simply naive to expect to be able to engage in a detached social science which is removed from the social or political context within which we operate. If researchers do not pay attention to the uses and implications for policy of their research then others will do it for them. Sociologists interested in any aspect of health may find their results used in the policy arena, whether they intended to do 'policy-relevant' research or not.

The organization of health policy research

There are, then, many incentives to be involved with research that is relevant to policy. How is such research organised? We could think of research happening within a three-way relationship

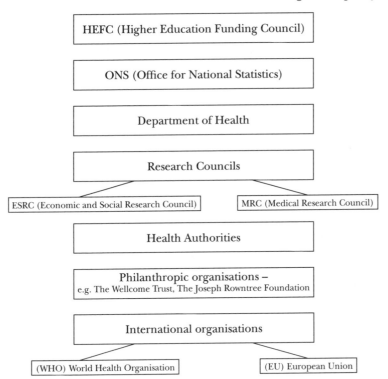

Figure 6.1 Who funds research for health policy?

between the client, who funds, or commissions, the research; the researchers, who actually carry it out; and those who are the subject of the research – the researched. These are not necessarily separate people or organisations, of course, but they often will be, and each might have very different ideas about what the research project is going to do for them.

The clients

To start with the clients: who does fund health policy research? Obviously this raises the question of how we define 'health policy research', but in terms of the broad definition used in this book, there are a number of organisations who commission and fund social science research for health policy. Some of them are listed in Figure 6.1.

The Office for National Statistics organises the 10-yearly census and the General Household Survey, which contain essential information for national and local health policy makers. The other organisations in Figure 6.1 fund others to do research. The HEFC funds such research indirectly, through its funding of the higher education sector which provides the institutional support (such as equipment and support staff) for many researchers. The Department of Health commissions research relevant to policy by inviting bids on topics which it has listed as priorities. It also funds some studies under schemes for 'responsive' funding, in which researchers apply to the regional offices. These will only be funded if the researchers can demonstrate that the results are likely to inform policy at some level. The research councils fund postgraduate studies (e.g. through PhD scholarships) as well as other research. They are more likely to fund theoretical work on policy, but the trend here has also been towards funding more 'applied' work (Newby 1993). The ESRC, for instance, invite bids for programmes of work relevant to particular policy questions. Some of these are in the health arena: between 1996 and 2000, for instance, the ESRC will be funding interdisciplinary work on socioeconomic health variations within the UK. Although the MRC is mainly concerned with medical research, rather than health policy, it does have an interest in multidisciplinary work in the area of health services and it does fund social research, including a Medical Sociology Unit in Glasgow.

Health authorities commission social science research to inform their own work of assessing local needs, prioritising service provision and evaluating local policy. Some of this is 'in house', carried out by public health departments (see Chapter 2) and some is commissioned from external researchers, both academics and (increasingly) market research companies. This kind of research is likely to be short-term and directed at answering specific policy questions. The case study in Box 6.1 is one example of this kind of work. Finally, philanthropic organisations such as the large charitable trusts and patient advocacy groups also fund some health policy research, although their contribution to the amount spent on research is quite small.

Researchers

The second group involved in the organisation of health policy research are the researchers, who include PhD students, employees of some of the organisations in Figure 6.1 and academics with an interest in health policy.

The first point to make is that the interests of those actually carrying out the research might not of course coincide with the clients. Caroline Wenger (1987), in her book on *The Research Relationship* outlines the very different models within which researchers and policy makers may be working. First, the very motivations for doing research may be quite different. For social researchers, there are the basic desires for academic credibility and furtherance of career, and the kinds of project that are most useful to policy makers are not necessarily the ones of most use as status symbols in the academic community, where practical research still has less status than theoretical research.

This difference is reflected in where research results are published. Time for writing up at the end of a project is often very limited, and the client may want the findings in a report that will reach those with political influence, rather than the academic journal which will improve the academic researcher's publication record. Publishing in peer reviewed academic journals is increasingly important now in institutes of higher education, where levels of funding rely to a large degree on how much and where members of a department have published over the last five years. Even more critical than the question of where to publish is the problem of unfavourable findings, which clients may not want published at all. The political needs of sponsors may act as a constraint on their ability to publish findings, or to publish them in a form acceptable to the researcher.

Another difference is time scale: researchers may not be used to adapting their methods to the short time scale needed for policy-relevant research, and feel that what they consider a 'rushed' study compromises academic credibility. Wenger is describing models of the different orientations of researchers and sponsors, and of course not all policy makers or all social researchers would share them. Her contrasting models do, though, give a general idea of some of the tensions that can arise. A good relationship between client and researcher can be achieved, Wenger says, but with careful negotiation: it cannot be taken for granted. Both the client and the researcher need successful research, for their own career advancement if not for any loftier social goals, although their professional orientations and institutional contexts may be very different. In the academic context, there is a high value placed on independence, creativity and autonomy, whereas the client – who is probably an administrator or manager – may work within an institutional context of hierarchy, loyalty and formal procedures.

Forging a working relationship, she suggests, entails first being explicit about the differences to foster debate and negotiation. Also necessary, she argues, is a more equal power status than that which exists at the moment, where those with the funds have all the power in a situation where there is little funding for basic social science. For a creative relationship, secure funding for researchers is needed, and academic freedom to pursue policy problems.

The case study in Box 6.1 is an example of health policy-orientated research which illustrates some of these issues, in a context where the relationship was a productive one.

Box 6.1 Using sociology to inform drug education policy

Background
Drug action teams are responsible for co-ordinating implementation of the national drug education policies within an area such as a county. In Kent, two health authority-based drug reference groups and three community drug reference groups feed information into, and disseminate information from, the drug action team. One, in West Kent Health Authority, wanted to inform their drug education policy for young people. Laura Hart and Neil Hunt, from Invicta Community Care NHS Trust (one of the trusts with contracts with the health authority), were commissioned to undertake a study of young people's perceptions of drug use. Their findings were reported in *Choosers not Losers?: Drug Offers, Peer Influences and Drug Decisions Amongst 11–16 year olds in West Kent*. This report, from Invicta Community Care, is an example of what is known as 'grey' literature: reports written primarily for an internal audience and not 'officially' published (i.e. it does not have an ISBN number, or a copy available in the British Library). As Hart and Hunt note in their introduction: 'It is assumed that readers will work in an area where drug prevention or drug education is part of their role . . . we have sought to avoid content which is exclusively of 'academic' interest' (Hart and Hunt 1997: 1). Their aim is to influence those who may be in a position to change policy, either strategically or in its implementation, rather than to influence academics.

The study
The study itself used different sociological methods, with a combination of focus groups (see discussion below) and interviews with young people, self-completed questionnaires and

observation. The methodological orientation was a humanistic and participatory one, which acknowledged the competence of the participants and attempted to reduce the hierarchy normally implicit in the researcher–researched relationship. The authors draw on the 'new sociology of childhood', which addresses the structural context of young people within society.

Just under half of the young people who participated had used drugs at least on an experimental basis, according to the questionnaire results, but qualitative data suggested that this was an underestimate, as many people talked about drug use in the more intimate context of a group discussion, but said they would not see themselves as 'users'. 'Drug offers' in practice were rather more complex than much drugs education assumes. Offers from strangers, such as dealers, are rare and easy to manage, but those from friends and siblings could be more problematic. However, 'peer pressure' was not really seen as a problem: young people choose their peers from those who share their lifestyle and attitudes, and drugs were not 'pushed' onto them, but were part of the general cultural life of young people.

Dissemination
The report will go out to those in a position to affect drug education in Kent: members of the Drug Reference Group, probation officers, teachers and health managers. Laura Hart and Neil Hunt are also hoping to write up aspects of the methodology and the findings for a more 'academic' audience, in peer-reviewed journals. Although these journals are not read widely by public sector managers, they are an important way in which research findings are disseminated more widely. They are also vital in terms of a research career. Many researchers are in short-term posts, employed on a contract just to carry out one study such as this one. Time for writing and dissemination is then very limited at the end of the contract. As well as writing the project report, dissemination may mean presenting it at meetings, talking to special interest groups and perhaps releasing information to the press. Choices have to be made about how to allocate time, and the 'academic' report may never get written. This can be a real problem for contract researchers, who are busy finding a new post at the very time when they also trying to write up the study. In academic departments, more credit is given for peer-reviewed publications than for experience disseminating project findings, and inevitably there is some trade-off between the two activities.

Source: Hart and Hunt 1997 and personal communications

To suggest that there are many agencies that *want* research is not to suggest that they will necessarily use the results of research, even if it is research that has been directly commissioned for some policy purpose, as was illustrated in Chapter 1 by the example of the Black Report on inequalities in health and the case study in Box 1.3 of the relationship between research and policy. However, there is a growing reliance on the part of both strategic and operational policy makers (such as the Department of Health and health authorities) on research findings, and it is likely that the skills of social researchers will continue to be needed.

The 'subjects' of health policy research

The last group involved in the organisation of research are the 'researched': those who are the subjects of health policy research. These could be patients, or health service professionals, or the community at large. These are the participants with the least power to define the research agenda, and there is considerable ethical debate about how the relationship between researchers and their subjects can be managed and what responsibilities researchers have to other participants in the research process.

Occasionally, the subjects of research are the clients who commission it. Williams and Popay (1994) discuss one example, arising from the Camelford poisoning incident in 1988, in which a lorry driver accidentally tipped 20 tons of aluminium sulphate into the water reservoir which served the town of Camelford in North Cornwall. Many members of the community and those who had been on holiday at the time reported a variety of symptoms that they attributed to the aluminium poisoning. The Department of Health commissioned its own research, from an expert committee, which perhaps predictably concluded that there were no long-term adverse effects from the water contamination. However, local people felt that their health had been adversely affected by the incident, and their response was to carry out their own research by monitoring the effects on their health. The different conclusions of the Department of Health's inquiry and the community's own research, argue Williams and Popay (1994), result from very different starting points about what counts as 'evidence', and sociology, they suggest, has a key role to play in developing methodologies which are sensitive to people's own definitions of health.

The more common relationship in research is perhaps where the 'researched' have the least power, in terms of defining the research question, directing the process of the research and deciding how the results are utilised. It has been noted that sociology has a tradition of being an advocate for the underdog: that sociologists have in general been more interested in the working classes than the aristocracy, in deviants rather than the police, or in factory workers rather than management. For Becker (1967) sociology had a role in challenging the 'hierarchy of credibility' that affords more legitimacy to elite versions of social reality (those from the top of their hierarchy), and, in his phrase, 'taking sides' was inevitable in doing research. Much of what has been written on the ethics and social responsibilities of researchers in the social sciences assumes that the research subjects will have less power in the relationship, but this is not always true in health policy research, where the 'subjects' may be those with considerable power over the policy agenda, such as NHS managers (Strong and Robinson 1990) or hospital consultants (Britten 1991).

Annette Lawson (1991) questions Becker's assumption that social scientists ought to 'take sides' in doing research. First, she argues, if sociology gains a reputation for being critical of medicine, then the credibility of findings is likely to be undermined and they are less likely to influence either medical practice or health policy. Second, she points to the very different political and economic climates of the 1960s, when Becker was writing about researchers' responsibilities, and the 1980s and 1990s, when academics are less likely to be in tenured posts and less able to get further funding if their research is deemed 'irrelevant' to the policy needs of the day. Lawson's third objection is that it is rather less clear than Becker suggested to identify the 'underdog' in health research. Her own example is from a study funded by a charity organised by patients with multiple sclerosis (MS), which supported a university-based research unit. Although as patients these participants were those at the bottom of most health service 'hierarchies of credibility', the size of this charitable organisation, which had a £3/4 million research budget, meant that they had in fact considerable power to dictate the process of the research, and affect the researcher's relationships with other participants, such as health professionals. When the organisation split, with some MS patients wanting to pursue different aims, the researchers' responsibilities were further split. In summary, Lawson maintains that the only justifiable and practical stance for researchers is one of independence from both sponsors and the subjects of the research, rather than 'taking sides'. Whether policy researchers take the view that research ought to strive for neutrality, or be explicit about its commitments to one version of social reality, they still have to consider the issue of research ethics: what their proper responsibilities are to those who participate.

Ethics

There are no hard and fast rules about ethical conduct in research, only frameworks which can orientate the researcher to consider the issues involved. Although it is essential to consider ethical issues to ensure that research does not contravene cultural norms about acceptable behaviour, ethics are not neutral principles but are rooted in social and political contexts. For instance, many such frameworks derive from models of medical research. An important early one covering medical experiments was the Nuremberg Code, which was drawn up after the Nuremberg trials of 1947 at which 23 Nazi doctors were accused of experiments on prisoners which included the deliberate infection of wounds with malaria and typhoid, the use of poisons and freezing of prisoners (Homan 1991). The Nuremberg Code outlined 10 principles:

1 Participation in experiments should be voluntary and the subjects fully appraised of the risks.
2 Medical experiments are only justified if they serve a humanitarian purpose that cannot be served by any other methods.
3 The likely outcomes should justify the risks involved.
4 The researchers should be thoroughly informed about risks before starting, with pilot studies on animals if appropriate.
5 Measures should be taken to avoid physical and psychological injury.
6 There can be no grounds for expecting the subject's death or disablement.
7 The researcher should take all possible precautions to avoid harmful effects.
8 Experimenters should be highly qualified and experienced.
9 The subjects should feel free to withdraw from an experiment, even when it is in progress.
10 The researcher should discontinue an experiment as soon as it is seen to cause undue harm or discomfort to a subject.

(Homan 1991)

In short, the researcher is seen to have a continuous duty to be concerned for the welfare of the subject: merely securing a one-off consent is not enough. Although some of the above tenets seem irrelevant to policy research (such as pilot studies on animals), many are important principles that still inform research ethics. Indeed, at first sight the code seems to be comprehensive and unambiguous, at least with regard to medical experiments, but there are some things not addressed which have been seen as important ethical issues in more recent years. What is considered 'ethical' changes historically, and also cross-culturally.

One issue that is now considered important is confidentiality. This concerns the right of subjects to have their identity disguised in any publications, and not to have information provided in a research context given to others. This is clearly an important issue for much health research, as we are often asking respondents to provide information that may not be in the public domain, such as experiences of encounters with health services or health care needs. It is also an important concern when doing research within health care settings when individual professionals may be providing information that could damage their relationships with others if made public, or damage the reputation of their organisation. Julienne Meyer, in the case study in Box 6.2, discusses this as a particular problem for action researchers.

Another issue not addressed by the Nuremberg Code, that would be of concern to health policy researchers, is that of publication and control over dissemination. To what extent do those who have given their time and knowledge as research subjects have the right to control what happens to that information? Should they be given the right to veto reports, for instance, before they are published?

Of course most policy research is not based on an experimental model, where some participants are subjected to an intervention, so in some senses codes covering medical research may seem less applicable to social research in the area of health policy. However, it cannot be assumed that methods such as interviewing or observation have no potential negative effects on subjects. Although those who do participate in research often report that it was on the whole a positive experience (Oakley 1990; Finch 1984), this is not inevitable, and possible distress needs to be considered. Securing informed consent to policy research may be more difficult than in medical experiments. In experimental designs, the researchers know at the start of the study what hypothesis they are testing, and what the likely outcomes are going to be. Many sociological studies of health policy are more exploratory, and the initial research question rather unspecific. Indeed, the research question may change as the result of early data collection. In these circumstances it is rather more difficult to inform participants fully of the likely outcomes and of what will happen to the results. Social science methods are rather more diverse than those used in medical research (some of the more common methods used in health policy research are listed below), and there is a greater variety of settings in which research is carried out. It is difficult to provide guidelines which will cover these disparate fields and methods of enquiry.

Many studies in health policy will have to be submitted to an ethics committee, which vets all research on patients. Local ethics committees assess the values and risks of the proposed study, along the kinds of criteria discussed. Different committees may use different guidelines, and any project looking at policy in more than one district may take some time to get approval. As these committees are primarily concerned with protecting patients from risks from medical experiments, they may be less skilled at reviewing proposals from social scientists involved in policy research, where the methodology may be very different to that of the randomised controlled trial seen as the method of choice in much medical research.

There are no comparative bodies for social science health policy research outside the health sector, although there are less formal mechanisms for ensuring that research is conducted in an ethical manner. One is the set of guidelines published by the British Sociological Association (BSA 1992), which begin with a statement about professional integrity: members are enjoined to strive for the freedom to research and publish and to do this 'accurately and truthfully'. The largest part of the BSA's code of ethics is taken up with relations with and responsibilities towards participants in research, noting that as researchers we enter into moral and personal relationships with those we study and that we have duties to them in thinking about the uses to which research findings will be put. The object of furthering knowledge does not entitle researchers to override the rights of others. They have obligations to ensure that participants give their informed consent and understand the extent of the agreed confidentiality and anonymity. For this reason, the BSA guidelines suggest that participant observation studies in which the role of the researcher is not revealed to those in the field ('covert' research) pose particular ethical problems. Although the data produced using these strategies may be more naturalistic, and less influenced by the presence of the researcher, it is not possible to secure informed consent. The study in Box 4.1 of access to GP services, in which the researchers presented themselves as potential patients, raises this issue. Whether the knowledge gained (which may not have been revealed using other methods) justified the lack of consent from health service staff to participation is a question to which there is no right answer.

One approach to research which attempts to restructure the power relations between the researcher and the researched is action research: a form of social experimentation in which a 'problem' is investigated in order to develop a possible strategy in solution. The action itself is taken, and then becomes part of the research, with research and setting interacting. Action research is premised on the notion that research ought to be with or for people, not on them (Reason 1988). Rather than viewing participants as 'research subjects', the researcher enters into a partnership, and the research is directed by all the participants. Action research aims to change, as well as just describe, the world. Box 6.2 summarises an example of action research from nursing, and Julienne Meyer's argument that rather than solving the ethical problems of research relationships with participants, action research raises its own particular issues.

Box 6.2 Using action research: an example from nursing practice

The issue: lay participation in care
Julienne Meyer was interested in lay participation in care on a hospital ward: the involvement of nonprofessionals in their own treatment and health maintenance. Although there is considerable support for lay participation in care, and nursing policy advocating 'partnerships' between patients and professionals, Meyer found few empirical studies of it being introduced in practice.

Methodology
Meyer's investigation of professional's attitudes to lay participation was carried out as action research. She joined a multidisciplinary team for one year, with the aim of facilitating lay participation in care and evaluating its implementation. The approach was 'nondirective', and aimed to enable participants to examine their own practice. The evaluation used a variety of methods including interviews, questionnaires and participant observation.

The findings

Although professionals were committed to the concept of lay participation (indeed they had volunteered to take part in this study of its implementation), there were many barriers to changing their own practice to involve patients. Interview data suggested that many professionals on the ward had reservations about whether lay participation was relevant to their own work. First, they were concerned about whether patients would feel that it was not their role to participate in care while they were in the hospital. Second, there were concerns about the legal implications. Third, involving patients was time-consuming, and on a busy ward (at a time of increasing workloads and low morale) extra work potentially increased stress. For medical staff, there were also concerns about patient involvement undermining the medical model. Observations suggested that patients had in fact little involvement in their own care. Meyer found that many of these barriers inhibiting change arose from problems in establishing good interprofessional teamwork on the ward. This was in part because of the high staff turnover (staff were often on the ward only for a short period, as part of their training, and had little time to find out about ward culture and organisation) and because of the domination of the team by medical professionals. Change in professional practice was unlikely to happen, argues Meyer, until health professionals developed more collaborative ways of working themselves.

Reflections on using action research

Meyer argues that action research might be a very useful approach for nursing, given the need both for reflections on practice which are accessible to practitioners and for a new epistemological approach which reflects the pluralism of the nursing profession. However, she cautions that it is not an 'easy' process. First, it can take considerable time to negotiate access to a site for the study, and then secure consent from all participants. Action research also poses different ethical problems from other approaches. Participants may be viewed as partners in the research process, but may find it harder to withdraw once they are involved. Within a large team, especially one which changes over the course of the project, it may be that some members are, or become, unwilling to take part in the project: should the researcher then leave, or is this an unethical waste of the effort of the enthusiastic members? The consent of managers may make it difficult for other staff to refuse to participate. It is also, argues Meyer, very difficult to alter the power imbalance between researcher and participant, even within an action research project. The researcher is likely to have power derived from academic knowledge, knowledge gained from talking in-depth to all participants in the field and from the position as ultimately an 'outsider' who will leave the field at the end of the study. In an action research project, the collaborative approach means that the information gained is likely to be deeper and more intimate, and the participant is therefore more likely to be at risk of betrayal and exploitation.

Sources: Meyer 1993a, 1993b

Analysing health policy from sociological perspectives involves, then, a set of issues similar to any other research activity. These include a consideration of who is funding the research, and why; who is doing the research and who is being researched. Because the arena of health policy is relatively diverse, researchers work in a range of settings, and the micro-politics of research organisation can be complex. The next section moves on from these considerations of organisation to macro-politics: the theoretical starting points, or assumptions, made about policy and how to analyse it.

Theoretical frameworks

'Theory' in policy research is often implicit. The assumptions researchers make about the forces shaping health policy, and their nature, are often not directly stated in reports or other publications. However, as we have already seen, theoretical and political perspectives affect both the policy agenda (that is, which issues become labelled as 'health policy concerns') and the range of responses that are considered. Thus, for instance, the rise of New Right thinking about welfare in the 1970s and 1980s made it possible to consider market solutions to the problems of rising costs in the NHS. Theoretical perspectives also affect how policy change is interpreted. The assumptions researchers make, both about how the world is and how it can be understood, shape the kinds of questions they ask, how they are asked and the types of knowledge produced as a consequence. Here, we outline some of the major theoretical traditions that influence policy analysts.

Marxist approaches to health policy

Marxist approaches are most evident in macro studies of the structure of health care systems, rather than micro studies of process.

One of the best known proponents is Vincente Navarro (1978, 1983), who has carefully articulated a Marxist analysis of the health sector and the role of the state within it. Health policy, for Navarro, is generated within class struggles, and can only be understood as part of the process of class conflict. Conventional histories of health policy in Britain, he argues, have suggested that 'progress' (for instance in establishing the welfare state) has happened because of the liberalism of the ruling classes. However, Navarro claims that policy shifts are the result of conflicts between different class interests in Britain. Following the industrial revolution in Britain, towards the end of the eighteenth century, the growing middle and working classes had, in some spheres, joint interests in challenging the still dominant power of the aristocracy. In the health sector this was reflected in demands from general practitioners and apothecaries (the healers of the middle and working classes, respectively) for a unified health profession with a monopoly of practice. Although resisted by the elite surgeons, this did happen in the 1858 Medical Act. The class origins of these sections of the profession still influence conflict within it today, claims Navarro, with the royal colleges enjoying more power and prestige within the profession than the general practitioners. Working-class militancy, which had grown with experience of strikes during the depression of the 1930s, was a key factor in demands for a nationalised health service just before the Second World War. Although the war itself delayed overt class conflict, it did lead to the state by necessity having a direct role in managing health services, for emergencies and to take care of the war wounded. The postwar election of 1945 was, claims Navarro, 'an arena for a battle between two competing forces – socialism and capitalism' (Navarro 1978: 38), embodied in the Labour and Conservative parties. The establishment of the NHS was hardly a revolutionary move, he argues, given the strong support in the country for a more radical proposal. Indeed, Bevan compromised with elite class interests in agreeing that hospital consultants could continue to do private practice, and he left the class basis of the profession intact.

Lesley Doyal (1979) is another writer who takes a Marxist approach to health policy. Doyal's approach is also one of examining the health care system as a way of understanding the wider social relations of capitalism: a sociology of policy, as well as a critical sociology for policy. She situates the problems of health and health care in modern society firmly within the profit motivation of capitalist production. Health and profit come into conflict, perhaps most visibly in areas such as health and safety legislation and pollution caused by industry. The needs of capitalist accumulation also affect health in less direct ways. The relative expense of wholemeal bread, for instance, is in the interests of large food multinationals, who mass produce poor quality bread with refined flour, which is consumed in greater bulk (because it is less filling) and provides 'by-products' such as bran which can be sold at more profit for animal feed. Marketing less nutritious products also opens up a new market for vitamins and health food supplements (Doyal 1979: 90–1). Capitalism produces a particular distribution of health and disease, in which those from poorer groups in society are most at risk (see Chapter 3) and it also produces specific social relations in medicine. The history of the NHS can only be understood if we ask who profits from it, and in whose interests it is organised.

Pluralist approaches

For Marxist analysts, power is a commodity which derives from access to the means of production, and it is held by one elite group in society, with the state acting in its interests. The content of health policy results from the conflicts between class interests, and the relative power of each class at a particular historical moment. Few policy analysts subscribe to this view: indeed Navarro (1983) has argued that the Marxist approach has been marginalised by writers on health, who have caricatured modern Marxist arguments and misrepresented their analytical power. In most writing on health policy, the assumptions about power are rather less explicit. Often policy is seen as being the result of compromises between different interest groups, who all have some influence over the shape of policy and can exercise some power. In this model, the pluralist position, any individual piece of policy making is the result of shifting coalitions between different groups which influence the process. No one elite is seen as invariably dominant, and the state is perceived to be more of a neutral arbiter of sectional views, rather than a defender of class interests. For the pluralists, the state in a liberal democracy supports the multiplicity of interests, and ensures that they are represented. As well as being a descriptive theoretical position for analysing health policy, pluralism is often used in a prescriptive way, claiming that this is how policy *ought* to be made. The liberal reformist perspective in policy making is one pluralist position.

Liberal reformist perspective

This is the status quo position. Most histories of the NHS are produced from within this perspective, although this is rarely made explicit. This view traces a 'progressive' account of the history of social development and reform throughout the first half of the twentieth century seen as culminating in the creation of the Welfare State in 1948. A liberal reformist perspective, made popular by the Fabian Society, suggests that incremental change and reform are the most productive way to produce social equality. More recently it has found expression in the various policies of Labour, Liberal and Social Democrat policies. In brief, it eschews any radical change (be it conservative or socialist) and suggests instead a more pluralist notion of competing interest groups, although recognising that some groups are more disadvantaged than others. In the early part of the twentieth century this position, formulated in the wake of Social Darwinism, also included the espousal of eugenic policies which aimed to increase the breeding of 'good stock' and to limit the breeding of genetically poor stock. This gave momentum to the family planning movement, as making contraception freely available to the 'feckless poor' was seen to be a way of implementing these strategies. Although the current widespread provision of family planning services appears to us as an outcome of 'liberal progress', the ideological antecedents are very different from currently acceptable values. This illustrates how what appears as 'liberal' in one political era can have entirely different connotations in another.

Of course the extremism of eugenic policies in Nazi Germany led this approach to be discredited. More recently, however, in response to the Black Report and to Margaret Whitehead's (1987) follow-up study *The Health Divide: Inequalities in Health in the 1980s*, explanations derived from 'sociobiology' have gained currency. This is a school of thought which suggests that social organisation, both in humans and animals, results from a combination of biological characteristics such as genetic constitution and population constraints, and that welfare, therefore, can only ameliorate certain inevitable social conditions (see, for instance, Wilson 1975 for an account of the sociobiologists' position). This approach has been usefully documented in Humphrey and Elford's (1988) critique of sociobiological explanations of the social class differences in infant mortality which followed the publication of Margaret Whitehead's work.

The discussion of the various explanations offered by the Black Report in Chapter 3 showed how different assumptions (such as whether biology or social environment causes inequality) have different implications for policy solutions.

A feminist perspective on welfare

What is a feminist perspective? A feminist perspective means taking gender into account. If Marxism is using 'class' as the analytic principle, feminism is using gender. What then is the gender-based view of welfare? A gender-based view of welfare considers the policies of 'welfare', that is, social policy and health policy, and asks how these policies affect women. What are the consequences of this policy for women? What does this policy tell us about the way women are viewed in society? Clearly, there is no single view or opinion on the answer to these questions; the interpretation will depend on the particular perspective from which they are viewed. This is equally true of feminism, as 'feminism' is not unitary and does not have a unitary perspective. There are many differing theoretical frameworks which underpin feminist analyses, for example, Marxist feminism, socialist feminism, liberal feminism, radical feminism, and lesbian feminism. More recently there have been Foucauldian analyses of gender, but as this calls into question the construction of the category 'women', we will leave it aside from the discussion here. Sometimes these perspectives are allied, for example in radical lesbian feminism; and sometimes their theoretical underpinnings are irreconcilable, for example, liberal feminism and Marxist feminism. What they do all share is the perception of women as a group who are structurally disadvantaged (that is, oppressed).

If we accept, for the time being at least, the notion of 'women as oppressed' we can see that the formulation of social policy is pertinent in a number of areas: health policies for example, which address reproduction and childbirth; the caring and control of bodies, (for example, child immunisation policies); dental checks or GP provision (where women are the predominant users of these facilities); social policies which determine welfare benefit levels (e.g. child benefits, single parent benefits) and childcare provision; economic policies which control the price and availability of food; these all impact on the majority of women in particular ways. A whole range of social policies produce 'normal women' and 'normal families' by sanctioning some living and working arrangements while penalising others (e.g. campaigns to support or discourage lone parents; allowing only married (not cohabiting) couples to adopt). Health, education and 'the family' are all crucial sites for the formulation of social policy, and all of these are crucial sites for women. They are gendered social spaces.

What becomes apparent, then, in the other theories of welfare is a lack: the *absence* of a gender perspective. Marxism, for example, excludes women from the analysis when they are not part of the 'labour process'. Traditionally, Liberalism excluded women because they were not 'sufficiently developed'. Fabians have addressed themselves to 'the woman question' but see this as a matter of change in social attitudes towards individuals and have little notion of women as a group. For the New Right, no social group can be taken into account as the unit of analysis is the individual; in a world based on market forces there can be no such thing as structured oppression. For Foucauldians 'women' is itself a socially constructed category and there can be no such thing as an essentialist notion of oppression.

This absence of theoretical attention itself speaks volumes. As we have seen, the crucial sites of welfare policies are centred on the accepted premise of gendered experience. This is particularly true of 'the family', a critical and central area for all state legislation, into which 'women' are subsumed. If, however, we accept for a moment the idea of 'women' as a coherent social group, a 'class', the possible outcomes of welfare legislation are similar to those proposed by the other theories; they can be reformist, functional, revolutionary or radical.

The liberal, reformist models are based on the notion that tinkering with the present system can make incremental changes culminating in the end point (hopefully not too far off) of equality. In the conflict models, health and social policy is seen to be produced by a social system which privileges and benefits men and, without radical change, will have no good outcomes for women. Indeed in these models healthcare becomes one site for resistance and opposition over issues such as childbirth, termination of pregnancy, donor insemination, and wages for housework, among others.

Feminism and social constructivism

As discussed in Chapter 2, there is yet another way of analysing health and other welfare policies, and that is to see them as constructing the categories which they then monitor and survey. This interpretation, as we have seen, suggests that 'social policy' acts as a system of regulation, as a means of ordering life and the social world, and that it takes as its object 'the family'. This view means that visible sanctions and punishments are no longer needed; instead, a system of regulatory beliefs and practices construct and reproduce our ideas about ourselves, our notions of what is normal. Crucial to this view then is that regulation takes place through normalisation. As outlined above, health and social policies act to produce and reproduce ideas about 'the family' (e.g. its presumed heterosexuality) and within this, create a particular view of women, an obscured view, an unarticulated view. This invisibility is such that even Foucauldian books on social policy do not identify a specifically gendered perspective (see, for example, Squires 1990).

To conclude, a feminist view means seeing the welfare world through gendered eyes. What one sees depends on one's vantage point, one's political disciplinary allegiances. A disciplinary perspective sees the advent of a 'social' policy as indicative of a new form of regulation, one that is based on normalisation and which focuses on 'the family'. In the same way that Smart (1992) documents the production of 'women' through the legal process, so we can examine the way in which 'women' are produced by welfare legislation and the implementation of health and social policies. For many sociologists, a constructivist perspective is potentially a sophisticated and analytical tool, but we have yet to render visible the construction of its gendered aspects.

The different theoretical assumptions made about how policy is or ought to be produced, and what its proper goals ought to be, clearly impact on how it is analysed. The next section of this chapter examines some of the methodological approaches available to those interested in both a sociology of policy and a sociology for policy.

Methodological approaches

As has been evident from the examples in this book, social science methods are used to investigate a range of health policy problems, from micro studies of policy implementation to macro studies of the development of health policy itself as an arena. When selecting a methodological approach, a first consideration is the kind of research question that is being addressed. One way of dividing up the kinds of questions that could be asked about health policy is to follow Donabedian (1976) and separate questions into those about outcome, those about process and those about structure. Outcome refers to the health change that has occurred as a result of health service intervention; process refers to the ways in which these interventions are delivered by people and organisations; structure refers to the organisation and funding of the health care system itself. Most recent social research in health policy has focused on aspects of process and outcome, rather than the structural level more often addressed by health economists and policy analysts. To illustrate, we address two contrasting areas in which sociology has been used to understand or aid health policy: eliciting users' views and needs (which contributes to understanding outcomes) and researching health services (examining the process).

In doing these kinds of research, a range of methodologies are available. It may be that the research question asks 'how many' or 'how often' a particular behaviour occurs (for example), thus implying a quantitative method; or it may be that the research question asks 'why' people believe or act as they do and 'what' they feel about it, implying a qualitative approach. Often a combination of the two is most useful. Similarly, a range of data collection techniques are available, although different methods are likely to be appropriate at different levels of analysis. The methods include randomised control trials, questionnaires, interviews, focus groups, participant observation and documentary analysis using a variety of population samples. The research may also take a number of design formats, for example, an experiment, a survey or a case study, each making different levels of analysis possible.

The following discussion gives examples of how these methodological approaches may be utilised in health policy research. It should be noted that not only will the research question and method be informed by the political background to the research but so will the way the findings are analysed and interpreted. For more detailed discussion of research methods and data analysis we refer the reader to the 'Further reading' section at the end of this chapter.

Eliciting users' views and needs

As has been discussed in previous chapters, a key issue in the provision of services is their planning and prioritisation (Chapter 3). In order to plan and deliver services, purchasers need to know what services are required. This presumes, implicitly or explicitly, a goal, for example, 'maximising health gain' or 'providing the most cost-effective service' or simply 'carrying on as before until the money runs out'. If, however, the goals (targets) are to be explicit, commissioners will have generally based these choices on their knowledge of the local conditions. This knowledge may well be the consequence of research. As discussed below, knowledge is not unproblematic, it is socially produced and validated, and, as we have seen in Chapter 2, research to assess need can take a number of different approaches depending on the outcome which is required. Thus methodological issues are crucially linked to the making of policy and to the kind of policy that is made.

Sampling

The first issue to be addressed is that of 'sampling'; that is, on which people will the research be based and how will they be selected? We saw in Chapter 2 how the new 'empowerment' model in health promotion has necessitated eliciting the views of potential or actual service users, and how potentially fraught this is.

Whole population samples do not, usually, mean including the total population but sampling from it in a *random* way, that is, ensuring that every person has an equal chance of being selected, for example, selecting every *n*th name from the electoral register. This presumes, however, that everyone will be registered on the electoral roll, which of course may not be the case, particularly for those who are homeless, refugees, seeking asylum or without legal residence. It would also exclude by default all those under voting age. Whole population sampling also presumes that the whole population are potential service users, whereas there may be sections of the population who would rarely, if ever, use the service in question (see Chapter 2 p. 55).

A random sample might also be selected from a particular segment of a whole population, say for example, from all those living within a certain health authority. It may be, however, that a sample population is required that is not random, but that can be said to be broadly similar to the majority of the population, that is, one that is *representative*, in which case certain criteria would need to be drawn up either to exclude those who were not representative or to include only those who were, for example, to ensure that all ethnic groups living in an area were represented in the research. Further, it would need to be ascertained whether these ethnic groups would need to be included in numbers proportionate to their percentage of the total population or whether it was desirable to have equal numbers of each group represented so that valid comparisons can be made between them. This might entail targeting certain groups, perhaps through local community associations. Sometimes a sample might be required which is representative of a particular characteristic, or stratum, of the population under scrutiny, such as women, or those on income support. This would mean selecting a *random stratified* sample. Defining the boundaries within which the sample will be chosen is called the *sampling frame*. Thus all sample populations, however selected, will be drawn from a sampling frame, that is, the defined parameters of the population from whom the sample is selected.

Data collection

Having defined an appropriate sampling frame, what techniques are available for eliciting the views of 'real people'? There are a number of methods, each producing different kinds of data. Perhaps most popular are surveys and questionnaires. These are easy to administer in large numbers and, provided they have been well designed, relatively easy to analyse. Questionnaires could be used, for instance, to ask hospital patients about the acceptability of services, or to ask young people about their health behaviour. Questionnaires can be postal or face to face, and again, the sample will be determined by the aims of the research. Public health departments have recently collaborated on 'lifestyle surveys' which ask questions about particular behaviours which relate to the *Health of the Nation* targets: they include questions about smoking, diet, exercise and so on and may be directed at particular population segments such as young people.

Another sampling technique is to ask the views of people in their capacity as the 'general public'. This takes the forms of a 'vox populi' survey, that is, approaching people in a public place (usually a high street or shopping area) and asking their views on a particular issue. It could be said then that these people are answering, not as particularly interested parties, but as the 'man or woman in the street'. These then most nearly approximate the 'common sense' view of the general population.

There has been some discussion in the methods literature regarding the distinction between 'public' and 'private' accounts (Cornwell 1984; Thorogood 1995; see also Box 2.4), that is, those views considered by the interviewee as 'publicly acceptable' and those more personal opinions which they would express only amongst those whom they felt had shared values. It has commonly been agreed that 'private' accounts are more likely to be expressed in in-depth interviews. These, however, require a great deal of 'researcher input', in both the execution and transcription. Social research interviews have, until recently, been one to one. Focus groups have, however, become a popular way of eliciting the views of people who share a common aspect of identity or experience. Focus groups involve a series of group discussions with different participants on the research theme. These are facilitated by the researcher who will have an interview guide but also be able to explore and follow up any new 'leads'.

This method has the advantage of allowing participants to react and interact with others like themselves, often leading to a development and clarification of research themes. When there is a gap in experience between the researchers and the subjects, the interactions within a focus group can provide a clear view of how others think and talk.

The method is also beneficial when investigating complex behaviour and motivations, as participants become more explicit about their own views as they hear others talk. They also illustrate that people are able to hold several contradictory views simultaneously. This can provide the researcher with insights into the range of opinions and the sets of circumstances that leads to one response rather than another. This methodology is also particularly appropriate when a friendly research method that is respectful and not condescending is needed. Focus groups are particularly effective where there is a power differential between participants and researchers as they provide a relatively safe space in which people can share their views. This makes focus groups a good way to sample hard-to-reach populations and can forge a human connection between those who commission a project and those who serve as the subjects of their investigations.

Combined uses of focus groups and sample surveys

Focus group methodology has the advantage of reaching larger numbers of a given population in a relatively short space of time compared to one to one interviews. But as with other qualitative research methods, the techniques can be used in conjunction with larger scale quantitative techniques. This may be before the main survey in order to facilitate questionnaire design, from the formulation of whole categories to the fine tuning of wording, or to anticipate survey nonresponse or refusal in hard-to-reach populations.

Focus groups can be used just after the survey with survey respondents to evaluate the survey process, for example, to ask about influences on the comprehension of survey questions and the subsequent responses. Focus groups can also be used after the survey results are analysed to corroborate findings or explore in greater depth the relationships suggested by quantitative analysis. Using focus groups concurrently with surveys can yield independent quantitative and qualitative research perspectives on the topics, which leads to a mutual enhancement of the analysis and understanding of each component by the other (a form of triangulation of the data) (Wolff *et al.* in Morgan 1993). One example of the use of focus groups to canvass user's views is Laxmi Jamdagni's account of a project in Bradford, in Box 6.3.

Box 6.3 An example of the use of focus groups to inform hospital policy

Context
This article was published in the wake of the death of Nasima Begum, the 11-year-old girl with a rare kidney disease who waited 53 minutes for an ambulance to take her from her east London home to the Royal London Hospital only three miles away. The author uses this tragic example to highlight the fear felt by many black and ethnic minority people that their race, ethnicity or culture will somehow impact on the quality of the treatment they receive in the NHS, fear that is not dispelled by changes to operations and management that do not address racism. Whilst fundamental inequalities in access to services and treatment remain, Jamdagni argues, the typical financial measures of efficiency, efficacy and economy cannot be a priority for black people.

The study
The purchaser/provider split has created the opportunity for services which are appropriate to the local community to be an explicit requirement. In this article Jamdagni reports on a Kings Fund initiative to support six health authorities in projects which develop services in collaboration with local communities.

One project took place in Bradford where approximately one fifth of the population are Asian (mainly from Pakistan). The project aim was to involve service users in identifying how services could be developed better to meet their needs in hospital. Interviews were held with recently discharged patients and focus groups run with local people. A number of aspects of the 'hotel' services were criticised, although the medical treatment itself was not. The aspect of the Asian meals service most commented on was the quality of the chapattis provided. There had been two previous attempts to provide appropriate and acceptable chapattis, one which involved training the hospital catering staff but which nevertheless resulted in the production of 'English style' Asian food. The second attempt had been to buy them in from an independent local supplier, but it was found that these became too hard after they were reheated in line with hospital requirements. The focus group interviews gave rise to the third solution: that was to purchase (employ) an in-house chapatti maker.

As Jamdagni notes, whilst to the health authority this was purchasing innovation, to the local people consulted it was an obvious solution, and one which they could have suggested much sooner if only they had been asked.

Source: Jamdagni 1994

Questions such as 'what health care needs do the local population have?' and 'what should this health authority prioritise in providing health services?' are questions primarily about *outcomes* of the health care system: what it produces, whether that is certain kinds of health care interventions or particular diets for inpatients. Methods such as surveys and focus groups have been utilised to aid local policy making on desirable outcomes, in providing information about the needs and views of populations. A second level of analysis is that of *process*: how the system is organised to produce these. When looking at process, other methods, particularly in-depth interviews and participant observation, have been used more often. This level of analysis looks at questions such as 'how have policy changes impacted on health service organisations?' or 'what are the processes by which policy is or is not implemented?'.

Researching health services

There have been many examples in this book of research which has addressed the organisation of health services, and the implementation of policy within the health sector, such as the study of single-handed GPs in Box 4.2 and the study of waiting list admissions in Box 5.3. Sociologists interested in how policy affects those delivering services, and how people working in the health care sector impact on policy, have used a variety of different methods, with qualitative methods such as in-depth interviews and participant observation being perhaps the most informative. Qualitative methods provide ways of exploring not only what people say they do, but also what they actually do in practice. They are primarily orientated towards *accounts* of the social world, and an interpretative understanding of what behaviour means in context. There has been considerable debate recently about the role of qualitative methods in health services research, with attempts to redress the balance towards quantitative methods apparent in scientific journals and the perceived 'higher status' of quantitative work. Qualitative methods have been seen as anecdotal, producing accounts which cannot be generalised or reproduced. Part of the response to these criticisms from sociologists working on health services has been to produce sets of criteria, which can be used by researchers, journal editors and readers to assess the worth of qualitative data (see, for instance, Mays and Pope 1996; Blaxter 1996; Boulton *et al.* 1996). These criteria address issues such as the selection of cases and participants (how was it justified? to what extent were they representative of others in the population?), the reliability of observations and coding (if there was more than one coder, how much agreement was there?), and the rigour of the analytical techniques used. They urge qualitative researchers to be transparent or explicit about the methods they use, in order that the reader can assess the value of the data produced.

Reference to criteria of reliability, validity and rigour do much to reassure those using qualitative research results that they are not merely the compilation of common sense or anecdotal accounts of processes within the health sector. However, the strengths of qualitative methods lie in their ability to reveal 'what is really going on', and move towards explanations for the patterns found in quantitative data. Catherine Pope's account of the process of constructing waiting lists, for instance, in Box 5.3, showed how the grounded practices of health workers shape the operation of policy, which would not have been revealed from an analysis of formal hospital policies, or a survey of staff. Techniques such as in-depth interviews also provide a way of accessing 'private' accounts of social reality, which may not be revealed in questionnaire surveys. The value of these 'private' accounts is that they may have more impact on behaviour than public ones (though this is not inevitable).

Qualitative methods also offer much for the sociologist of health policy. Questions such as 'how is management achieved?' can be addressed through examining the talk of key actors, on the assumption that it is through talk that we construct the social world. Thus, the study of emergency admissions in Box 5.2 showed how the rhetorics of professionals constructed the reality and legitimacy of bed management and the hospital as an organisation. Similarly, Michael Traynor, using some of the techniques of discourse analysis, examined the language used by health service managers in new Community Trusts (Traynor 1996). His approach was to see transcripts of interviews with managers as 'texts' which could then be analysed to deconstruct the discourses evident. Managers, he argued, utilised discourses of measurement and control to establish their rationality as privileged over that of others, and so achieve stable meaning within what would otherwise be an unstable and uncertain organisation.

To argue for the value of qualitative methods for a sociology for and of health policy does not imply that quantitative methods are of little use in looking at process in health services. Archie Cochrane (1972), who argued passionately for outcomes to be tested through randomised controlled trials (RCTs), has also been cited as legitimising the use of RCTs as the 'gold standard' for evaluating process. RCTs are experiments in which those receiving the intervention and those not are randomly assigned to the different groups, ideally without those involved in the process of providing the intervention or coding its results knowing which group the participants were in. Because participants are randomly assigned, any significant differences in results between those in the experimental group (who receive the intervention) and in the control group (who don't) are assumed to be as a result of the intervention itself. Although sociologists have not, on the whole, used RCTs in health policy research, there have been some calls for their greater utilisation. Ann Oakley (1990), for instance, argues that they may be the method of choice if the researcher wants to demonstrate that some aspect of process does have an effect on outcome. Further, carrying out an RCT can be a useful way of questioning assumptions about health care. Her own example is from a study of social support in pregnancy, which was assumed, but not proved, to predict better outcomes, such as lower risk of a low birthweight baby. Although there were problems with using an RCT design to test this assumption (such as resistance from research midwives, whose professional ideology supported providing interventions on the basis of need, rather than random allocation), Oakley argues that there were clear benefits in using this method. Random allocation, for instance, demonstrated that sometimes the perceptions of professionals about a woman's 'need' for extra social support were wrong. Also, the results of an RCT are much more likely to persuade policy makers of the value or otherwise of an intervention.

Conclusion: the politics of knowledge

As the earlier discussion of theoretical and methodological approaches makes clear, 'knowledge' is not unproblematic. What we 'know' and what research 'finds out' is produced by the social and political context. Currently, valid 'knowledge' is, in the main, constituted by 'scientifically' proven 'facts' rather than, for example, astrological predictions or religious tenets. What is rarely acknowledged, however, is that this 'scientific knowledge' is also a product of its social context.

'Science', like any other explanatory system, is not a given, located somewhere 'out there'. It does not pre-exist the social (see Chapter 2). It follows that 'scientific research' is equally a product of social forces and cannot, therefore, be epistemologically separate and 'objective'. There is a tendency, though, to reify science by making it appear as something outside of society. But 'science' is not a 'thing' with an objective identity, it is rather a set of practices which are a human sociocultural product. The concept of 'scientific research' is however, so taken for granted that those involved barely see it as a process at all (for a fuller discussion of these ideas see Thorogood 1997b).

This has important consequences for the development of policy which is frequently justified on the grounds of (scientific) evidence. What 'Scientific research' is done and how the results impact on policy is influenced by all manner of social and political considerations. At the political level, for example, the UK tobacco industry has until now spent about £100m a year on advertising which generated around £18 million in tobacco product tax and VAT for the Treasury. In contrast the government has spent well under £10 million on antismoking campaigns (figures from Customs and Excise Annual Report 1994/5, quoted in the ASH factsheet 1995). At a cultural level, the research projects most likely to get financial backing are those which appear to have some utilitarian purpose and that do not undermine too radically the current received wisdom (Potter and Mulkay 1982). There are also ways in which the individual researcher unavoidably brings values to the research process. For example, as we have seen, the choice of research topic and hypothesis, the method of observation, data analysis and interpretation of data, the choice of co-workers and the way in which any findings are made known will all affect the outcome and subsequent conclusions drawn from a project.

Scientific research, then, is a product of the economic, social and political interests of the time. But 'science' itself is a paradigm; that is it is only one of potentially many explanatory systems, both historically and in contemporary use, which may seem or have seemed equally plausible and legitimate (after all people who believed the earth was flat also thought they knew the truth). In news stories, for example, 'experts' called in to make sense of events for the lay population are frequently scientists or medics, not priests or astrologers, at least when called to explain the physical world. But this is a relatively recent development: science is a product of the Enlightenment, the age of reason (see also Chapter 2). This 'paradigm shift' occurred approximately 200 years ago moving from *teleological* (purposive) to *rational* (progressive/scientific) explanatory frameworks (Kuhn 1962). Scientific medicine (and modern dentistry) are discourses (practices and explanations) produced by this philosophy. This perspective suggests that science is just another paradigm. There is no *a priori* reason why one paradigm should be superior to another (see Chalmers 1982 for a fuller discussion of the Kuhnian notion of paradigms). Science, in this way of thinking, is a cultural product. Scientific projects arise from particular 'ways of seeing' (Berger and Luckmann 1967). They are carried out by researchers who already know which questions to ask (or more particularly, which *not* to ask). Scientists are not, for example, trying to prove scientifically how many angels we can get on the head of a pin.

Kitzinger (1986) identifies several strategies which contribute to the maintenance of this position of dominance. In one, which she labels 'mythologies of expertise', 'lay' is contrasted with 'expert' knowledge. This distinction acts to construct science as the source of legitimate knowledge. This does, of course, have implications for the making of health policy in that, as noted earlier in this chapter, quantitative research methods are often deemed to produce data which are more 'real' (hard data) than those produced by qualitative methods (soft data) along with all the concomitant gendered implications of these terms.

Scientific research's claim to being 'value free', at least in its execution, is dependent upon its methodological claims. Critiques of research findings often point to methodological failings or omissions. Claims to scientific method are intended to imply some special type of merit or reliability, to mark out valid from invalid knowledge, and this is what distinguishes it from other ways of making predictions about the world. However, this reliance on methodological claims implies the uniform acceptance of scientific method's underlying principles and in that respect, it is little different from the claims made by (for example) the Azande about their system of witchcraft (Evans Pritchard 1937). This scientific methodology, therefore, has an implicit epistemology: it starts from the assumption that things exist independent of the act of perception. This is often demonstrated by the use of visual imagery in the language of research such as 'shedding light', 'opposing perspectives', 'myopic/short-sighted/blind'. This suggests that the invisible is made visible, that 'reality' is exposed for all to see, 'proving', therefore, that science is not *socially* constructed.

Finally, scientific validity is also claimed by reference to external sources, for example, the use of references and the use of statistics, as we have done throughout this book. As we mentioned in Chapter 2, producing statistical analyses is a relatively recent practice. Again, our familiarity with these techniques usually obscures the social nature of their production. For example, 'Pearson's correlation' was subject to a great deal of contention and debate during the nineteenth century when the mathematical basis for this calculation was disputed by Frances Galton, who had produced a completely different way of testing for the significance of a correlation.

Sociology can not only provide useful insights into the practices of medical and dental science for practitioners (see for instance Scambler 1991; Helman 1985; Clarke *et al.* 1996; Burke and Croucher 1996), but is also able critically to appraise the practices of both science and medicine as social systems themselves: that is, it is both a 'sociology *for*' and 'sociology *of*', and this brief appraisal of scientific research as a cultural practice forms part of the latter. What then are the implications for health policy? Perhaps most significantly this approach calls into question the whole rationale for 'evidence-based medicine', which has been central to much recent health care policy (see for instance Audit Commission 1994 and NHSME 1996 for policy on using evidence-based medicine to improve prescribing practice). After all, when claims are made for the 'evidence base' of something, it is presumed that the 'evidence' is unproblematic. We are now in a position to query what 'evidence' is produced and by whom? What is the 'evidence' being used to prove or support? As sociologists of science point out, the technical superiority of a new product or service as demonstrated in scientific research is not a sufficient – or even necessary – condition of it being disseminated and widely adopted (Greer 1988, 1994). Instead, what some sociologists (Latour 1987; Prout 1996) have called an 'actor-network' has to be mobilised, which includes both human and nonhuman actors. Once a network has reached a point at which it has stabilised, in that it has a discrete and unified form, then claims for the legitimacy of a new technology can be made. There are no pre-existing scientific facts: claims have to be made for them, and successful claims are the result of social, rather than just technical, processes (Mulkay 1979). One such process is that of peer review: gaining the approval of others in the discipline, so that results are published, then cited widely in order to become 'facts' and part of the body of knowledge of a discipline (see, for instance, Latour and Woolgar 1986). Another is the cultural shifts which make it possible for scientists to ask the questions they do, and produce particular kinds of knowledge. Jackson (1995), for instance, examines the ways in which new cultural 'styles' in thinking about bodies (that, for instance, they are interdependent, and that biochemical markers are a scientifically acceptable way of inferring behaviour) made it possible for researchers to look at the health risks of passive smoking as a legitimate area of investigation. In a similar vein, Green (1997) examines the emergence of a distinct knowledge about accident prevention in the middle of the twentieth century, as the result of shifting cultural discourses about risk and expert knowledge. Once the scientific credibility of such knowledge is established, it can be utilised as 'evidence' for policy.

Our discussion of differing theoretical perspectives showed how they can be used to analyse the production of health policy. Taking a social constructionist perspective on the production of knowledge allows a critical approach to the rationale used to justify policies and to the research on which they are based. Thus, as noted above, the prevailing political ideology will strongly influence the type of policies implemented, and indeed those issues which are considered in need of 'health policy'.

Exercise

Academic journals that publish articles reporting empirical research findings related to health policy include:

> *Sociology of Health and Illness*
> *Social Science and Medicine*
> *International Journal of Health Services*
> *Health Education Journal*
> *Health Policy*
> *Journal of Health Politics, Policy and Law*
> *Health and Place*
> *Health and Social Care in the Community*

Survey one or more of the recent volumes of these journals for a paper reporting research that was of or for health policy and write a critical review of the article. Some of the issues you may want to consider are:

> What methods were used, and what was the rationale for them?
> Identify the main players, i.e. funder, client, researcher, subjects.
> Are there any pertinent ethical issues which the researchers have (or should have) addressed?
> Are there identifiable 'ideological' frameworks? Are any apparent by their absence? (e.g. Marxism, feminism)?
> Are there implicit assumptions of neutrality (e.g. that 'economics' does not have a political dimension)?
> What are the implications, if any, of the findings for health policy?

Further reading

There are a large number of good general textbooks on social science research methods. They include:

May, T. (1993) *Social Research: Issues, Methods and Process*, Milton Keynes: Open University Press;

Harvey, L. and McDonald, M. (1993) *Doing Sociology: A Practical Introduction*, London: Macmillan;

Gilbert, N. (1993) *Researching Social Life*, London: Sage;

Harvey, L. (1990) *Critical Social Research*, London: Allen and Unwin.

The most comprehensive and readable book on ethics is Homan, R. (1991) *The Ethics of Social Research*, London: Longman.

Those which are orientated specifically towards research in the health field include:

McConway, K. (ed.) (1994) *Studying Health and Disease*, Buckingham: Open University Press.

This book is part of the Open University's excellent Health and Disease series. Although the focus is in studying health, rather than policy, the approach to different methods (including epidemiology, history, survey research and qualitative sociology) is a useful one for a student researcher of health policy.

Mays, M. and Pope, C. (1996) *Qualitative Research in Health Care*, London: BMJ Publishing Group.

Clearly written, very practical guide to using qualitative methods in health research, taken from articles in the *British Medical Journal*. Written for a sceptical audience, the chapters here also present the case for qualitative methods.

Popay, J. and Williams, G. (ed.) (1994) *Researching the People's Health*, London: Routledge.

Overview chapters of the role of research in the post-1990 reforms NHS, and interesting case studies of research for needs assessment and outcomes in health policy, and of users' involvement in health research.

On theoretical approaches to policy analysis, the following is useful:

George, V. and Wilding, P. (1994) *Welfare and Ideology*, Brighton: Harvester Wheatsheaf.

A clear introduction to a range of ideologies and their implications for welfare policy. Includes a chapter on feminism.

Appendix: The National Health Service (NHS)

During the Second World War, there was considerable public support for a health care system which provided universal coverage, to replace the patchwork of health provision which existed in Britain. The 1911 National Insurance Act had extended general practice services to working men, but large sections of the population were not covered and the voluntary hospitals were in financial difficulties. A Labour government was returned with a large majority in 1945, with a commitment to establishing a welfare state. Aneurin Bevan was the Minister for Health who negotiated the NHS Act 1946, which established Britain's National Health Service in 1948. It was the world's first collectivised health care system. Funded from general taxation, the NHS nationalised the local authority and voluntary hospitals and provided universal, comprehensive health care for the whole population, free at the point of delivery. It was originally a 'tripartite' system with primary care, hospital and public health functions under different management structures. Local authorities maintained control over the public health and community services, and 'family practitioner' professionals (GPs, GDPs, pharmacists and opticians) continued as independent contractors, administered by executive councils. Hospitals were managed by hospital management committees which were responsible to a regional hospital board.

The form of the new system was the result of compromises between different interests, and Klein (1995) has argued that dilemmas inherent in the creation of the NHS continue to provide problems for planners and policy makers. One constraint was the organisation of the new system, which had to balance public control with local autonomy. Local authorities already had the structures for managing some health services, and would have been perhaps an obvious choice to manage the new system, but separate health authorities were established, partly to maintain central control. However, the lack of coterminosity (shared boundaries) with local authorities continues to cause difficulties for health managers and workers at all levels. A second dilemma was Bevan's inability to control the medical profession. In the hospital sector, consultants were permitted to continue private practice as well as NHS employment, and dominated management of the NHS at all levels. Funding was a further problem: despite adding prescription charges, other charges and National Insurance contribution as additional revenue to that from taxation, the NHS inherited antiquated hospital stock and ever-increasing costs, and continued, according to many analysts, to be underfunded.

The NHS was reorganised in 1974, when the tripartite structure was, to some extent, unified and joint consultative committees were set up to enable health and local authorities jointly to plan services for those in need of community care. Area health authorities (AHAs), which (apart from those in London) shared boundaries with both local authorities and family practitioner committees (which replaced the executive councils), were created as a new tier of administration. Below these were district health authorities (DHAs). The 1974 reorganisation also introduced community health councils to represent consumer views.

Financial issues dominated the NHS during the 1970s, as economic growth stopped and Britain entered a recession. Political debate centred on how to fund a service apparently in permanent 'crisis', as costs escalated. The NHS was reorganised again in 1982, when AHAs were replaced with smaller DHAs in an effort to decentralise and simplify the levels of bureaucracy. Conservative policies for the NHS during the 1980s stressed both management and responsiveness to the consumer. The Griffiths Report of 1983 advocated that a system of general management should be introduced to the NHS, to replace the 'consensus management' that was dominated by medical interests. Competitive tendering was introduced in 1983, when health authorities were required to put catering, laundry and domestic services out to tender and accept the most competitive contract.

By the end of the 1980s, the Conservative prime minister Margaret Thatcher had announced a wide-ranging review of the NHS, which informed the 1989 White Paper *Working for Patients*. Although this left the principles of the NHS unchanged (it continued to be financed through taxation and was free at the point of delivery) it did radically change the structure. The 'commissioning' functions, such as deciding on health care needs and monitoring how they are met, were left with the health authorities, whereas the 'providing' functions were administratively separate in the hospital and community trusts, which had self-governing status. In addition, large GP practices could hold their own budgets for some secondary care services. Although the review did not identify extra funds for the NHS, the resulting 'internal market' was intended to drive down expenditure through competition between providers. Despite the intention of devolving control to individual commissioning authorities, the reforms have had the effect of both centralising control of the NHS with the Department of Health and also potentially fragmenting the service, as commissioners can contract with a range of providers. It has proved difficult to monitor the extent to which the internal market has changed the way health services are delivered in practice, as the reforms are only one set of changes to the service over the last few years, no routine research was built into the process, and the time scale for evaluation has been short (Robinson and Le Grand 1994). Figure A.1 shows the main elements of the NHS in 1991, after the reforms. Since then, Regional Health Authorities have been abolished, and DHAs and FHSAs have merged to commission all primary and secondary care services for their populations. Figure A.2 shows the structure of the NHS in 1996.

There are many histories of the NHS available. One of the best is Rudolf Klein's (1995) *The New Politics of the National Health Service* (3rd edn), London: Longman. From a Marxist perspective, Vincente Navarro (1978) *Class Struggle, the State and Medicine*, London: Martin Robertson, examines the establishment and history of the NHS up to the 1970s. The further reading in Chapter 1 also has some books on British health policy over the last 50 years.

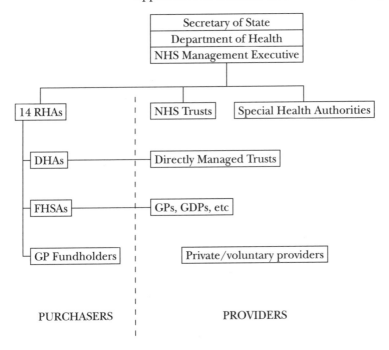

Figure A.1 The structure of the NHS following the 1990 reforms

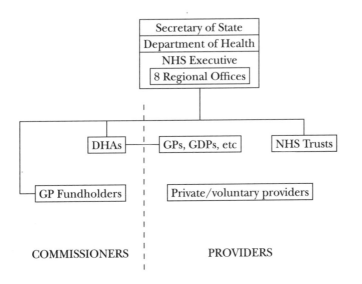

Figure A.2 Structure of the NHS 1996

References

Acheson, Sir D. (Chair) (1988) *Public Health in England. The Report of the Committee of Inquiry into the Development of Public Health Function*, London: HMSO.

Ackerknecht, E. (1967) *Medicine at the Paris Hospital 1794–1848*, Baltimore, MD: Johns Hopkins University Press.

Acton, T. and Chambers, D. (1990) 'Where was sociology in the struggle to re-establish Public Health?', In P. Abbott and G. Payne (eds) *New Directions in the Sociology of Health*, Basingstoke: Falmer.

Adams, J. (1995) *Risk*, London: UCL Press.

Ahmad, W.I.U. (1993) *'Race' and Health in Contemporary Britain*, Buckingham: Open University Press.

Allen, C.D., Barker, T., Newton, J.T. and Thorogood, N. (1992) 'Public perceptions of the funding of NHS dental services', *British Dental Journal*, 173: 175–6.

Allsop, J. (1990) *Changing Primary Health Care: The Role of Facilitators*, London: King's Fund Centre.

Allsop, J. (1995) *Health Policy and the NHS: Towards 2000*, London: Longman.

Allsop, J. and May, A. (1993) 'Between the devil and the deep blue sea: managing the NHS in the wake of the 1990 Act', *Critical Social Policy* 13: 5–22.

Andrews, A. and Jewson, N. (1993) 'Ethnicity and infant deaths: the implications of recent statistical evidence for materialist explanations', *Sociology of Health and Illness* 15: 137–55.

Armstrong, D. (1983) *Political Anatomy of the Body*, Cambridge: Cambridge University Press.

Armstrong, D. (1985) 'Space and time in British general practice', *Social Science and Medicine* 20: 659–66.

Armstrong, D. (1993) 'Public health spaces and the fabrication of identity', *Sociology* 27: 393–410.

ASH (1995) *ASH Factsheet No 3*, November. London: ASH.

Ashley, F.P. and Allen, C.D. (1996) 'Oral health promotion', in J.J. Murray (ed.) *Prevention of Oral Disease*, Oxford: OUP.

Ashton, J. and Seymour, H. (1988) *The New Public Health*, Milton Keynes: Open University Press.

Atkinson, P. (1981) *The Clinical Experience: The Construction and Reconstruction of Medical Reality*, Farnborough: Gower.

Audit Commission (1986) *Making a Reality out of Community Care*, London: HMSO.

Audit Commission (1994) *A Prescription for Improvement: Towards More Rational Prescribing in General Practice*, London: HMSO.

Audit Commission (1996) *What the Doctor Ordered: A Study of GP Fundholders in England and Wales*, London: HMSO.

Balarajan, R. and Raleigh, V.S. (1990) 'Variations in perinatal, neonatal, postnatal and infant mortality in England and Wales by mother's country of birth 1982–1985', in M. Britton (ed.) *Mortality and Geography*, OPCS Series DS no 9. London: HMSO.

Balint, M. (1957) *The Doctor, his Patient and the Illness*, London: Tavistock.

Barron, S. (1995) 'Mouth almighty', *Time Out*, Nov 22–29: 32–3.

Bartley, M. (1994) 'The relationship between research and policy: the case of unemployment and health', in A. Oakley and A.S. Williams (eds) *The Politics of the Welfare State*, London: UCL Press.

Beck, U. (1992) *Risk Society: Towards a New Modernity* (tr. R. Ritter), London: Sage.

Becker, H. (1967) 'Whose side are we on?', *Social Problems* 14: 239–47.

Berger, P. and Luckmann, T. (1967) *The Social Construction of Reality*, Harmondsworth: Penguin.

Berridge, V. and Thom, B. (1996) 'Research and policy: what determines the relationship?' *Policy Studies* 17: 23–34.

Birch, S. (1986) 'Increased patient charges in the National Health Service: a method of privatising primary care', *Journal of Social Policy* 15: 168.

Blane, D., Davey Smith, G. and Bartley, M. (1993) 'Social selection: what does it contribute to social class differences in health?', *Sociology of Health and Illness* 15: 1–15.

Blaxter, M. (1990) *Health and Lifestyles*, London: Routledge.

Blaxter, M. (1996) 'Criteria for the evaluation of qualitative research papers', *Medical Sociology News* 22(1): 68–71.

Blinkhorn, A. (1979) 'Behavioural sciences in the dental curriculum', *British Dental Journal*, 147: 117–20.

Bloor, M. and McIntosh, J. (1990) 'Surveillance and concealment: a comparison of techniques of client resistance in therapeutic communities and health visiting', in S. Cunningham Burley and N. McKeganey (eds) *Readings in Medical Sociology*, London: Tavistock/ Routledge.

BMA (British Medical Association) (1990) *The BMA Guide to Living with Risk*, Harmondsworth: Penguin.

Boulton, M., Tuckett, D., Olson, C. and Williams, A. (1986) 'Social class and the general practice consultation', *Sociology of Health and Illness* 8: 325–50.

Bowler, I. (1993) ' "They're not the same as us": midwives' stereotypes of South Asian descent maternity patients', *Sociology of Health and Illness* 15: 157–78.

Boulton, M., Fitzpatrick, R. and Swinburn, C. (1996) 'Qualitative research in health care: II. A structure review and evaluation of studies', *Journal of Evaluation in Clinical Practice* 2: 171–9.

Bradshaw, J. (1972) 'A taxonomy of social need' in G. McLachlan (ed.) *Problems and Progress in Medical Care: Essays on Current Research*, Oxford: Oxford University Press.

Britten, N. (1991) 'Hospital consultants' views of their patients', *Sociology of Health and Illness* 13: 83–97.

Bryan, B., Dadzie, S. and Scafe, S. (1985) *The Heart of the Race*, London: Virago.

BSA (British Sociological Association) (1992) 'BSA guidelines for good professional conduct and ethical practice', *Sociology* 26: 609–707.

Bulmer, M. (ed.) (1982) *The Uses of Social Research*, London: Allen and Unwin.

Bunton, R. and Burrows, R. (1995) 'Consumption and health in the "epidemiological" clinic of late modern medicine', in R. Bunton, S. Nettleton, and R. Burrows (eds) *The Sociology of Health Promotion*, London: Routledge.

Burchell, G., Gordon, C. and Miller, P. (1991) *The Foucault Effect: Studies in Governmentality*, London: Harvester Wheatsheaf.

Burke, L. and Croucher, R. (1996) 'Criteria of good dental practice generated by general dental practitioners and patients', *International Dental Journal*, 46: 3–9.

Bury, M. and Gabe, J. (1990) 'Hooked? Media responses to tranquillizer dependence', in P. Abbott & G. Payne (eds) *New Directions in the Sociology of Health*, Brighton: Falmer Press.

Calnan, M. (1988) 'Images of general practice: the perceptions of the doctor', *Social Science and Medicine* 27: 579–86.

Calnan, M., Cant, S. and Gabe, J. (1993) *Going Private: Why People Pay for their Health Care*, Milton Keynes: Open University Press.

Castel, R. (1991) 'From dangerousness to risk', in G. Burchell, C. Gordon and P. Miller (eds) *The Foucault Effect: Studies in Governmentality*, Hemel Hempstead: Harvester Wheatsheaf.

Chadwick, E. (1842) *Report on the Sanitary Conditions of the Labouring Population of Great Britain*. Reprinted (1965) by M.W. Flinn (ed.) Edinburgh: Edinburgh University Press.

Chalmers, A.F. (1982) *What is this Thing Called Science?*, Milton Keynes: Open University Press.

Charlton, J. (1996) 'Which areas are the healthiest?' *Population Trends* 83, Spring: 17–24.

Clarke, M., Locker, D., Murray, H. and Payne, B. (1996) 'The oral health of disadvantaged adolescents in North York, Ontario', *Canadian Journal of Public Health, Revue Canadienne de Sante Publique*, 87: 261–3.

Cochrane, A.L. (1972) *Effectiveness and Efficiency*, London: Nuffield Provincial Hospitals Trust.

Cohen, S. (1973) *Folk Devils and Moral Panics*, London: Paladin.

Colhoun, H. and Prescott-Clarke, P. (1996) *Health Survey for England 1994*, London: HMSO.

Consumers' Association (1992) *Which? Way to Health*, July. London: Consumers' Association.

Cornwell, J. (1984) *Hard-earned Lives*, London: Tavistock.

Costongs, C. and Springett, J. (1997) 'Joint working and the production of a City Health Plan: the Liverpool experience', *Health Promotion International* 12: 9–18.

Coulter, A. (1995) 'Shifting the balance from secondary to primary care', *British Medical Journal* 311: 1447–8.

Critical Public Health (1992) *Drains, Dustbins and Diseases*, 3(3).

Dalley, G. (1996) *Ideologies of Caring*, London: Macmillan.

Danziger, R. (1996) 'Compulsory testing for HIV in Hungary', *Social Science and Medicine* 43: 1199–204.

Davey Smith, G., Bartley, M. and Blane, D. (1990) 'The Black Report on socio-economic inequalities in health 10 years on', *British Medical Journal* 301: 373–7.

Davies, C. and Rosser, J. (1986) *Processes of Discrimination: A Study of Women Working in the NHS*, London: HMSO.

Davison, C., Davey-Smith, G. and Frankel, S. (1991) 'Lay epidemiology and the prevention paradox: the implications of coronary candidacy for health education', *Sociology of Health and Illness* 13: 1–19.

DHSS (Department of Health and Social Security) (1976) *Prevention and Health: Everybody's Business*, London: HMSO.

DHSS (Department of Health and Social Security) (1980) *Inequalities in Health*, London: HMSO.

DHSS (Department of Health and Social Security) (1983) *NHS Management Inquiry Report (Griffiths Report)*, London: DHSS.

DHSS (Department of Health and Social Security) (1987) *Promoting Better Health*, London: HMSO.

DHSS (Department of Health and Social Security) (1988) *Community Care: An Agenda for Action*, London: HMSO.

DOH (Department of Health) (1989) *Caring for People*, Cmnd. 7615, London: HMSO.

DOH (Department of Health) (1992) *The Health of the Nation: A Strategy for Health in England*, London: HMSO.

DOH (Department of Health) (1995) *A Policy Framework for Commissioning Cancer Services*, London: HMSO.

DOH (Department of Health) (1996) *Health and Personal Social Service Statistics for England*, London: The Stationery Office.

Dingwall, R. and McIntosh, J. (eds) (1978) *Readings in the Sociology of Nursing*, Edinburgh: Churchill Livingstone.

Dixon, J. and Welch, H.G. (1991) 'Priority setting: lessons from the Oregon Experiment', *The Lancet* 337: 891–4.

Donabedian, A. (1976) *Some Issues in Evaluating the Quality of Health Care*, Kansas City: ANA Publications.

Donovan, J.L. (1984) 'Ethnicity and health: a research review', *Social Science and Medicine* 19: 663–70.

Donzelot, J. (1980) *The Policing of Families: Welfare Versus the State*, London: Hutchinson.

Dopson, S. and Waddington, I. (1996) 'Managing social change: a process-sociological approach to understanding organisational change within the National Health Service', *Sociology of Health and Illness* 18: 525–50.

Douglas, M. (1986) *Risk Acceptability According to the Social Sciences*, London: Routledge and Kegan Paul.

Downer, M., Gelbier, S. and Gibbons, D.E.G. (1994) *Introduction to Dental Public Health*, London: FDI World Dental Press.

Doyal, L. (with Pennell, I.) (1979) *The Political Economy of Health*, London: Pluto Press.

Doyal, L. and Gough, I. (1991) *A Theory of Human Need*, London: Macmillan.

Doyal, L. (1993) 'The role of the public in health care rationing', *Critical Public Health* 4: 1:52.

Drever, F., Whitehead, M. and Roden, M. (1996) 'Current patterns and trends in male mortality by social class (based on occupation)', *Population Trends* 86 (Winter 96): 15–21.

Durkheim, E. (1963) *Suicide: A Study in Sociology*, London: Routledge and Kegan Paul.

Egbert, L., Battit, G., Welch, C. and Bartlett, M. (1964) 'Reduction of post-operative pain by encouragement and instruction of patients', *New England Journal of Medicine* 270: 25–6.

Elston, M.A. (1991) 'The politics of professional power: medicine in a changing health service' in J. Gabe, M. Calnan and M. Bury (eds) *The Sociology of the Health Service*, London: Routledge.

Enthoven, A.C. (1985) *Reflections on the Management of the National Health Service*, Occasional Paper no 5. London: Nuffield Provincial Hospitals Trust.

Evans Pritchard, E. (1937) *Witchcraft, Oracles and Magic among the Azande*, Oxford: Clarendon Press.

Etzioni, A. (1967) 'Mixed scanning: a "third" approach to decision making', *Public Administration Review* 27: 385–92.

Ewald, F. (1991) 'Insurance and risk' in G. Burchell, C. Gordon, and P. Miller (eds) *The Foucault Effect: Studies in Governmentality*, Hemel Hempstead: Harvester Wheatsheaf.

Finch, H., Keegan, J. and Ward, K. (1988) *Barriers to the Receipt of Dental Care – A Qualitative Study*, London: Social and Community Planning Research.

Finch, J. (1984) ' "It's great to have someone to talk to": ethics and the politics of interviewing women', in C. Bell and H. Roberts (eds) *Social Researching: Politics, Problems, Practice*, London: Routledge.

Finch, J. (1986) *Research and Policy: The Uses of Qualitative Methods in Social and Educational Research*, Brighton: Falmer Press.

Fitzpatrick, R., Hopkins, A. and Warvard-Watts, O. (1983) 'Social dimensions of healing', *Social Science and Medicine* 17: 501–10.

Foucault, M. (1976) *The Birth of the Clinic*, London: Tavistock.

Foucault, M. (1979) *Discipline and Punish, the Birth of the Prison*, Harmondsworth: Penguin.

Freeborn, D.K. and Pope, C.R. (1994) *Promise and Performance in Managed Care: The Pre-paid Group Practice Model*, Baltimore, MD: Johns Hopkins University Press.

Freidson, E. (1970) *Profession of Medicine: A Study of the Sociology of Applied Knowledge*, New York: Dodd Mead.

Gantley, M., Davies, D.P. and Murcott, A. (1993) 'Sudden infant death syndrome: links with infant care practices', *British Medical Journal* 306: 16–20.

Gavilan, H. (1992) 'Care in the community for older housebound people: institutional living in your own home?' *Critical Public Health* 3: 14–18.

Glennerster, H., Matsangis, M. and Owen, P. (1994) *Implementing GP Fundholding: Wild Card or Winning Hand*, Buckingham: Open University Press.

Goffman, E. (1961) *Asylums*, Harmondsworth: Penguin.

Gordon, I., Lewis, J. and Young, K. (1977) 'Perspectives on policy analysis', *Public Administration Bulletin* 25: 26–30.

Graham, H. (1986) *Caring for the Family*, Research Reports no 1, London: Health Education Council.

Graham, H. (1987) 'Women's smoking and family health', *Social Science and Medicine* 25: 47–56.

Gray, H. (1962) *Anatomy: Descriptive and Applied* (33rd edition, edited by D.V. Davies and F. Davies). London: Longman.

Green, J. (1993) 'The views of single handed general practitioners: a qualitative study', *British Medical Journal* 307: 607–10.

Green, J. (1996) 'Time and space revisited: the creation of community in single handed British general practice', *Health and Place* 2: 85–94.

Green, J. (1997) *Risk and Misfortune: A Sociology of Accidents*, London: UCL Press.

Green, J. and Armstrong, D. (1993) 'Controlling the "bed state": negotiating hospital organisation', *Sociology of Health and Illness* 15: 337–52.

Green, J. and Armstrong, D. (1995) 'Achieving rational management: bed managers and the crisis in emergency admissions', *The Sociological Review* 43: 743–64.

Greer, A.L. (1988) 'The state of the art versus the state of the science: the diffusion of new medical technologies into practice', *International Journal of Technology Assessment in Health Care* 4: 5–26.

Greer, A. (1994) 'Scientific knowledge and social consensus', *Controlled Clinical Trials* 15: 431–6.

Grundy, E. (1996) 'Population review: (5) The population aged 60 and over', *Population Trends* 84: 14–20.

Gustafsson, U. and Nettleton, S. (1992) 'The health of two nations: national strategies for public health and health promotion in England and Sweden', *International Journal of Sociology and Social Policy*, 12(3): 1–25.

Haggard, L. (1996) 'Hospital at home', in P. Gordon and J. Hadley (eds) *Extending Primary Care*, Oxford: Radcliffe Medical Press.

Ham, C.J. (1981) *Policy Making in the National Health Service*, London: Macmillan.

Harrison, S. (1995) 'NHS organisation: reassembling the jigsaw', *Critical Public Health* 6: 5–19.

Hart, L. and Hunt, N. (1997) *Choosers not losers?: Drug Offers, Peer Influences and Drug Decisions Amongst 11–16 year olds in West Kent*, Maidstone: Invicta Community Care NHS Trust.

Hawkes, G. (1995) 'Responsibility and irresponsibility: young women and family planning', *Sociology* 29: 257–73.

Helman, C. (1985) *Culture, Health and Illness*, Bristol: Wright.

Hensher, M., Fulop, N., Hood, S. and Ujah, S. (1996) 'Does hospital-at-home make economic sense? Early discharge versus standard care for orthopaedic patients', *Journal of Royal Society of Medicine* 89: 548–51.

Higgins, J. (1988) *The Business of Medicine: Private Health care in Britain*, London: Macmillan Education.

Hinton, T. (1994) 'Researching homelessness and access to health care', *Critical Public Health* 5(3): 33–8.

Hogwood, B. and Gunn, L. (1984) *Policy Analysis for the Real World*, Oxford: Oxford University Press.

Homan, R. (1991) *The Ethics of Social Research*, London: Longman.

Honigsbaum, F. (1985) 'Reconstruction of general practice: failure of reform', *British Medical Journal* 290: 823–6.

Hughes, D. (1989) 'Paper and people: the work of the casualty reception clerk', *Sociology of Health and Illness* 11: 392–408.

Humphrey, C. and Elford, J. (1988) 'Social class differences in infant mortality: The problem of competing hypotheses', *Journal of Biosocial Science* 20: 497–504.

Hunt, S. (1989) 'The public health implications of private cars', in C.J. Martin and D.V. McQueen (eds) *Readings for a New Public Health*, Edinburgh: Edinburgh University Press.

Hunter, D.J. (1993) 'Rationing and health gain', *Critical Public Health* 4(1): 27–33.

Hunter, D.J. (1994) 'From tribalism to corporatism: the managerial challenge to medicine', in J. Gabe, D. Kelleher, and G. Williams (eds) *Challenging Medicine*, London: Routledge.

Jackson, P. (1995) 'The development of a scientific fact: case of passive smoking', in R. Bunton, S. Nettleton and R. Burrows (eds) *The Sociology of Health Promotion*, London: Routledge.

Jamdagni, L. (1994) 'Purchasing for black populations: some local and national indicators for improved access and quality', *Critical Public Health* 5: 14–23.

Jewson, N.D. (1976) 'The disappearance of the sick-man from medical cosmology, 1770–1870', *Sociology* 10: 225–44.

Johnson, N. (1990) *Reconstrucing the Welfare State: A Decade of Change 1980–1990*, Hemel Hempstead: Harvester Wheatsheaf.

Johnson, T. (1995) 'Governmentality and the institutionalisation of expertise', in T. Johnson, G. Larkin and M. Saks (eds) *Health Professions and the State in Europe*, London: Routledge.

Jones, J. and Cameron, D. (1984) 'Social class analysis: an embarrassment for epidemiology', *Community Medicine* 6: 37–46.

Kaye, C.F. and West, C.R. (1986) 'Change and understanding', *Hospital and Health Services Review* 82: 252–3.

Kitzinger, C. (1986) *The Social Construction of Lesbianism*, Sage: London.

Klein, R. (1995) *The New Politics of the NHS*, London: Longman.

Kuhn, T. (1962) *The Structure of Scientific Revolutions*, Chicago: Chicago University Press.

Labour Party (1997) Election Manifesto, London: Labour Party.

Lalonde, M. (1974) *A New Perspective on the Health of Canadians*, Ottawa: Minister of Supply and Services.

Lam, T. and Green, J. (1994) 'Primary health care and the Vietnamese community: a survey in Greenwich', *Health and Social Care* 2: 293–9.

Lambeth, Southwark and Lewisham Health Commission (1995) *The Future of Primary Care in South East London*, London: LSL Health Commission.

Latour, B. (1987) *Science in Action*, Cambridge, MA: Harvard University Press.

Latour, B. and Woolgar, S. (1986) *Laboratory Life: The Construction of Scientific Fact*, Princeton, NJ: Princeton University Press.

Lawler, J. (1991) *Behind the Screens: Nursing, Somology and the Problem of the Body*, Edinburgh: Churchill Livingstone.

Lawson, A. (1991) 'Whose side are we on now? Ethical issues in social research and medical practice', *Social Science and Medicine* 32: 591–9.

Le Grand, J. (1991) *Equity and Choice*, London: Harper Collins.

Le Grand, J. and Bartlett, W. (1993) *Quasi Markets and Social Policy*, London: Macmillan.

Light, D. (1994) 'Assessing the US health reforms', *Medical Sociology News* 19: 22–5.

Lindblom, C. (1959) 'The science of muddling through', *Public Administration Review* 39: 517–26.

Lipsky, M. (1980) *Street Level Bureacracy: Dilemmas of the Individual in Public Service*, New York: The Russell Sage Foundation.

Littlejohns, P. and Victor, C. (1996) *Making Sense of A Primary Care Led Health Service*, Oxford: Radcliffe Medical Press.

London Health Planning Consortium (1981) *Primary Health Care in Inner London* (Acheson Report), London: London Health Planning Consortium.

Lupton, D. (1995) *The Imperative of Health*, Sage: London.

Mays, N. and Pope, C. (eds) (1996) *Qualitative Research in Health Care*, London: BMJ Publishing Group.

Macfarlane, J.K. (1977) 'Developing a theory of nursing: the relation of theory to practice, education and research', *Journal of Advanced Nursing*, 2: 261–70.

Marmot, M.G., Rose, G., Shipley, M., and Hamilton, P.J.S. (1978) 'Employment grade and coronary heart disease in British civil servants', *Journal of Epidemiology and Community Health* 32: 244–9.

Marmot, M.G., Davey Smith, G., Stansfield, S., Patel, C., North, F. and Hend, J. (1991) 'Health inequalities among British civil servants: the Whitehall II study', *Lancet* 337: 1387–93.

Martin, C. (1988) 'How do you count maternal satisfaction? A user-commissioned survey of maternity services', in H. Roberts (ed.) *Women's Health Counts*, London: Routledge.

McKeown, T. (1979) *The role of Medicine: Dream, Mirage or Nemesis?*, Oxford: Blackwell.

Means, R. and Smith, R. (1994) *Community Care: Policy and Practice*, London: Macmillan.

Mechanic, D. (1991) 'Sources of countervailing power in medicine', *Journal of Health Politics, Policy and Law* 16: 485–206.

Mechanic, D. (1995) 'Dilemmas in rationing health care services: the case for implicit rationing', *British Medical Journal* 310: 1655–9.

Meyer, J. (1993a) 'New paradigm research in practice: the trials and tribulations of action research', *Journal of Advanced Nursing* 18: 1066–72.

Meyer, J. (1993b) 'Lay participation in care: a challenge for multidisciplinary teamwork', *Journal of Interprofessional Care* 7: 57–66.

Mills, C. Wright (1959) *The Sociological Imagination*, Oxford: Oxford University Press.

Morgan, D. (ed) (1993) *Successful Focus Groups*, London: Sage.

Morley, V., Evans, T., Higgins, R. and Lock, P. (1991) *A Case Study in Developing Primary Care: The Camberwell Report*, London: King's Fund Centre.

Morris, J. (1993) *Independent Lives? Community Care and Disabled People*, London: Macmillan.

Mort, F. (1987) *Dangerous Sexualities: Medico – Moral Politics in England Since 1830*, London: Routledge and Kegan Paul.

Morton, S. (1992) 'Public health medicine and local authorities', *Critical Public Health* 3(3): 40–48.

Mulkay, M. (1979) *Science and the Sociology of Knowledge*, London: George Allen and Unwin.

Navarro, V. (1978) *Class Struggle, the State and Medicine: An Historical and Contemporary Analysis of the Medical Sector in Great Britain*, London: Martin Robertson.

Navarro, V. (1983) 'Radicalism, Marxism and medicine', *International Journal of Health Services* 13: 179–202.

Nettleton, S. (1991) 'Wisdom, diligence and teeth: discursive practices and the creation of mothers', *Sociology of Health and Illness* 13: 98–111.

Nettleton, S. (1992) *Power, Pain and Dentistry*, Buckingham: Open University Press.

Nettleton, S. (1995) *The Sociology of Health and Illness*, Cambridge: Polity Press.

Nettleton, S. and Harding, G. (1994) 'Protesting patients', *Sociology of Health and Illness* 16: 38–61.

Newby, H. (1993) 'Social science and public policy', *RSA Journal* May: 365–72.

NHSME (National Health Service Management Executive) (1996) *Primary Care: The Future*, London: The Stationery Office.

The Nuffield Report (1993) *Education and Training of Personnel Auxiliary to Dentistry*, The Nuffield Foundation: London.

Oakley, A. (1990) 'Who's afraid of the randomised controlled trial?: some dilemmas of the scientific method and "good" research practice', in H. Roberts (ed.) *Women's Health Counts*, London: Routledge.

Offe, C. (1984) *Contradictions of the Welfare State*, London: Hutchinson.

Office of Health Economics (OHE) (1995) *Compendium of Health Statistics*, London: Office of Health Economics.

ONS (Office for National Statistics) (1997) *Living in Britain: Results from the 1995 General Household Survey*, London: The Stationery Office.

Office of Population Censuses and Surveys (OPCS) (1994) *1991 Census: Economic Activity Great Britain*, vol. 2, London: HMSO.

Oliver, M. (1993) 'Disability and dependency: a creation of industrial societies?', in J. Swain, V. Finkelstein, S. French, and M. Oliver (eds) *Disabling Barriers – Enabling Environments*, London: Sage.

O'Malley, P. (1992) 'Risk, power and crime prevention', *Economy and Society* 21: 252–73.

Oswald, N. (1989) 'Why not base clinical education in general practice?' *The Lancet* July 15th: 148–9.

Pape, R. (1978) 'Touristry: a type of occupational mobility', in R. Dingwall and J. McIntosh (eds) (1978) *Readings in the Sociology of Nursing*, Edinburgh: Churchill Livingstone.

Pearson, M. (1986) 'Racist notions of ethnicity and culture in health education', in S. Rodmell and A. Watt (eds) *The Politics of Health Education*, London: Routledge and Kegan Paul.

Pelling, M. (1983) 'Medicine since 1500', in P. Corsie and P. Weindling (eds) *Information Sources in the History of Science and Medicine*, London: Butterworth.

Plant, M. and Plant, M. (1993) *Risk Takers: Alcohol, Drugs, Sex and Youth*, London: Routledge.

Pollock, A.M. (1993) 'Rationing – implicit, explicit or merely complicit?' *Critical Public Health* 4(1): 19–23.

Pope, C. (1991) 'Trouble in store: some thoughts on the management of waiting lists', *Sociology of Health and Illness* 13: 192–212.

Potter, J. and Mulkay, M. (1982) 'Making theory useful: utility accounting in social psychologists' discourse', *Fundamenta Scientae* 3: 259–78.

Prior, L. (1991) 'Mind, body and behaviour: theorisations of madness and the organisation of therapy', *Sociology* 25: 403–21.

Prior, P. (1995) 'Surviving psychiatric institutionalisation: a case study', *Sociology of Health and Illness* 5: 651–67.

Prout, A. (1996) 'Actor network theory, technology and medical sociology: an illustrative analysis of the metered dose inhaler', *Sociology of Health and Illness* 18: 198–219.

Putnam, R.D., Leonardi, R. and Nanetti, R.Y. (1993) *Making Democracy Work: Civic Traditions in Modern Italy*, Princeton, NJ: Princeton University Press.

Rees Jones, I. (1992) 'Oregon, public health and social control', *Critical Public Health* 3(2): 12–16.

Registrar General (1839) *Annual Report of Births, Marriages and Deaths*, London: HMSO.

RCGP (Royal College of General Practitioners) (1972) *The Future General Practitioner: Learning and Teaching*, London: RCGP.

Reason, P. (1988) *Human Inquiry in Action: Developments in New Paradigm Research*, London: Sage.

Richardson, R. (1989) *Death, Dissection and the Destitute*, Harmondsworth: Pelican.

Roberts, H., Smith, S. and Bryce, C. (1993) 'Prevention is better . . .', *Sociology of Health and Illness* 15: 447–63.

Roberts, H., Smith, S. and Lloyd, M. (1992) 'Safety as social value; a community approach', in S. Scott, G. Williams, S. Platt & H. Thomas (eds) *Private Risks and Public Dangers*, Aldershot: Avebury.

Robinson, R. and Le Grand, J. (eds) (1994) *Evaluating the NHS Reforms*, Hermitage: Policy Journals/King's Fund Institute.

Rocheron, Y. (1988) 'The Asian Mother and Baby Campaign: the construction of ethnic minorities' health needs', *Critical Social Policy* 22: 4–23.

Rodmell, S. and Watt, A. (1986) *The Politics of Health Promotion: Raising the Issues*, London: Routledge and Kegan Paul.

Rogers, A. and Pilgrim, D. (1995) 'The risk of resistance: perspectives on the mass childhood immunisation programme', in J. Gabe (ed.) *Medicine, Health and Risk*. Oxford: Blackwell.

Rose, N. (1990) *Governing the Soul: The Shaping of the Private Self*, London: Routledge.

Saks, M. (1994) 'The alternatives to medicine', in J. Gabe, D. Kelleher, and G. Williams (eds) *Challenging Medicine*, London: Routledge.

Sankar, S. (1988) 'Patients, physicians and context: medical care in the home', in M. Lock and D. Gordon (eds) *Biomedicine Examined*, Dordrecht: Kluwer.

Salvage, J. (1985) *The Politics of Nursing*, London: Heinemann Nursing.

Savage, J. (1987) *Nurses, Gender and Sexuality*, London: Heinemann Nursing.

Scambler, G. (ed.) (1991) *Sociology as applied to medicine* (3rd edition), London: Ballière Tindall.

Scull, A.T. (1977) *Decarceration: Community Treatment and the Deviant. A Radical View*, Englewood Cliffs, NJ: Prentice Hall.

Scull, A.T. (1983) 'Madness and segregative control: the rise of the insane asylum', in P. Brown, (ed.) *Mental Health Care and Social Policy*, London: Routledge and Kegan Paul.

Secretary of State for Health (1989) *Working for Patients*, Cmnd 555, London: HMSO.

Seward, M. and McEwen, E. (1987) *The Provision of Dental Care by Women Dentists in England and Wales in 1985: A Ten Year Review*, London Hospital Medical College Dental School, Crown Copyright.

Simon, J. (1988) 'The ideological effects of actuarial practices', *Law and Society Review* 22: 772–800.

Small, N. (1989) *Politics and Planning in the National Health Service*, Milton Keynes: Open University Press.

Smart, C. (1992) *Regulating Womanhood: Historical Essays on Marriage, Motherhood and Sexuality*, London: Routledge.

Smith, D. (1980) *Overseas Doctors in the National Health Service*, London: Policy Studies Institute.

Smith, P. (1992) *The Emotional Labour of Nursing*, London: Macmillan.

Squires, P. (1990) *Anti-Social Policy. Welfare Ideology and the Disciplinary State*, Hemel Hempstead: Harvester Wheatsheaf.

Stacey, M. (1988) *A Sociology of Health and Healing*, London: Unwin Hyman.

Stacey, M. (1991) 'Medical sociology and health policy: an historical overview', in J. Gabe, M. Calnan, and M. Bury (eds) *The Sociology of the Health Service*, London: Routledge.

Stocking, B. (1992) 'The introduction and costs of new technologies', in E. Beck, S. Lonsdale, S. Newman, and D. Peterson (eds) *In the Best of Health?* London: Chapman and Hall.

Strauss, A., Schatzman, L., Ehrlich, D., Bucher, R. and Sabshin, M. (1963) 'The hospital and its negotiated order', in E. Freidson (ed.) *The Hospital in Modern Society*, New York: Free Press of Glencoe.

Strong, P. and Robinson, J. (1990) *The NHS: Under New Management*, Milton Keynes: Open University Press.

Thorogood, N. (1992) 'You pays your money and takes your choice', *Sociology of Health and Illness* 14: 23–37.

Thorogood, N. (1995) 'London dentist in HIV scare: HIV and dentistry in popular discourse', *Primary Dental Care* 2(2): 59–60.

Thorogood, N. (1997a) *Constructing Ethnic Identities Through Oral Health Behaviours: Findings from Focus Groups*, Paper given to the BSA Medical Sociology Conference, York.

Thorogood, N. (1997b, in press) 'Questioning science', *British Dental Journal* 182.

Tones, B.K. (1986) 'Health education and the ideology of health promotion: a review of alternative approaches', *Health Education Research* 1(1): 3–12.

Townsend, P. and Davidson, N. (1982) *Inequalities in Health: The Black Report*, Harmondsworth: Penguin.

TP-NET (Total Purchasing National Evaluation Team) (1997) *Total Purchasing: A Profile of National Pilot Projects*, London: King's Fund Publishing.

Traynor, M. (1996) 'A literary approach to managerial discourse after the NHS reforms', *Sociology of Health and Illness* 18: 315–40.

Tucker, D. (1991) 'Letter', *British Medical Journal* 303: 362.

Tuckett, D., Boulton, M., Olson, C. and Williams, A. (1985) *Meetings between Experts: An Approach to Sharing Ideas in Medical Consultations*, London: Tavistock Publications.

UKCC (United Kingdom Central Council for Nursing, Midwifery and Health Visiting) (1986) *Project 2000: A New Preparation for Practice*, London: UKCC.

Walker, M. (1988) 'Training the trainers: socialisation and change in general practice', *Sociology of Health and Illness* 10: 282–302.

Warwick, I., Aggleton, P. and Homans, H. (1988) 'Constructing commonsense – young people's beliefs about AIDS', *Sociology of Health and Illness* 10: 213–33.

Weber, M. (1949) *The Methodology of the Social Sciences*, New York: Free Press.

Webster, C. (ed.) (1993) *Caring for Health: History and Diversity*, Buckingham: Open University Press.

Wenger, G.C. (1987) *The Research Relationship: Practice and Politics in Social Policy Research*, London: Allen and Unwin.

Whitehead, M. (1987) *The Health Divide: Inequalities in Health in the 1980s*, London: Health Education Council.

Whitfield, M. and Bucks, R. (1988) 'General practitioners' responsibilities to their patients', *British Medical Journal* 297: 398–400.

Wilkinson, R.G. (1989) 'Class mortality differentials, income distributing and trends in poverty 1921–1981', *Journal of Social Policy* 18: 307–35.

Wilkinson, R.G. (1992) 'Income distribution and life expectancy', *British Medical Journal* 304: 165–8.

Wilkinson, R.G. (1996) *Unhealthy Societies: The Afflictions of Inequality*, London: Routledge.

Williams, A. (1985a) 'Economics of coronary artery bypass grafting', *British Medical Journal*, 291: 326–9.

Williams, A. (1987) 'Measuring quality of life: a comment', *Sociology* 21: 326–9.

Williams, S. and Calnan, M. (1991) 'Key determinants of consumer satisfaction with general practice', *Family Practice* 8: 237–42.

Williams, G. and Popay, J. (1994) 'Researching the people's health: dilemmas and opportunities for social scientists', in J. Popay and G. Williams (eds) *Researching the People's Health*, London: Routledge.

Willis, A. (1996) 'Commissioning: the best for all', in P. Littlejohns and C. Victor (eds), *Making Sense of a Primary Care Led Health Service*, Oxford: Radcliffe Medical Press.

Wilson, E.O. (1975) *Sociobiology*, Cambridge, MA: Harvard University Press.

World Health Organisation (1978) *Report of the International Conference on Primary Health Care, Alma Ata 1977*, Geneva: WHO.

World Health Organization, Europe (1985) *Targets for Health For All*, Copenhagen: WHO.

World Health Organisation, Health and Welfare, Canada, Canadian Public Health Association (1986) *Ottawa Charter for Health Promotion*, WHO, Copenhagen.

Zola, I. (1978) 'Medicine as an institution of social control', in J. Ehrenreich (ed.) *The Cultural Crisis of Modern Medicine*, New York: Monthly Review Press.

Index